Arielle Essex is a leading speaker, trainer and consultant. After years of experience in complementary medicine (osteopathy, kinesiology and naturopathy), she trained extensively in Neuro-Linguistic Programming, hypnosis and emotional intelligence before founding her own business.

Based in London, Arielle is Director of Practical Miracles, an NLP training company devoted to guiding people to reach their full potential for success and happiness. She has been creating and delivering transformational seminars in Europe and the Middle East since 1988.

Praise for *Compassionate Coaching*:

'Arielle Essex is a consummate teacher. Now she shares her gifts of charity, healing and grace in a way in which we can all take part. Her book is a treat for the soul.'
    Chuck Spezzano Ph.D., author of *Happiness is the Best Revenge*

'Don't just read this book – study it. *Compassionate Coaching* is a powerful self-coaching guide full of useful techniques and inspiration for living the life you want.'
    Robert Holden Ph.D, author of *Shift Happens!*

'Arielle has done a fabulous job of blending spiritual and psychological insights with down-to-earth practicality to create a potent recipe for true happiness and success.'
    Nick Williams, author of *The Work We Were Born to Do*

'A personal and inspiring account of healing and the steps people can take in order to help heal themselves . . . a powerful roadmap for change that can be followed by anyone who desires to bring more health and healing into their lives. I highly recommend it.'
    Robert Dilts, author of *From Coach to Awakener*

Compassionate Coaching

How to Heal Your Life and
Make Miracles Happen

Arielle Essex

RIDER
London . Sydney . Auckland . Johannesburg

9 10

Published in 2004 by Rider, an imprint of Ebury Publishing.

Ebury Publishing is a Random House Group company.

The Random House Group Limited Reg. No. 954009

Addresses for companies within the Random House Group can be found at www.randomhouse.co.uk

A CIP catalogue record for this book is available from the British Library.

ISBN 9781844132362

Penguin Random House is committed to a sustainable future for our business, our readers and our planet. This book is made from Forest Stewardship Council® certified paper.

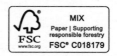

Printed and bound in Great Britain by Clays Ltd, Elcograf S.p.A.

This book is dedicated to my mother with love.

Contents

Preface

Compassionate Coaching aims to deliver self-coaching techniques that anyone can use. When you need to change, improve relationships, or heal old wounds, wouldn't it be useful to have an experienced guide to show you the way? This book outlines a thorough approach to help direct your journey and make your dreams a reality. Whether you need to completely overhaul your life, or just make a few small changes, the steps to success are easy to follow.

Standard coaching offers useful one-to-one guidance, encouragement, and support to help teach you the strategies to achieve specific goals. But a coach can't be inside your head twenty-four hours a day. Ultimately you need your own internal compass, so you can keep yourself on course. You need to learn how to channel your energies in the right direction. You need to be well grounded before you can leap to new heights.

The intention of this book grew out of many years teaching and working with thousands of clients. You can learn from the experience of others, reading the many case studies that describe some of the pitfalls and traps to avoid along the way. Each chapter carefully assists you in preparing yourself for each stage, before you make the next move. You can learn how to strengthen your positive qualities and remove the obstacles from your path.

Someone who has travelled the path before and knows the way makes the best guide. Self-coaching means learning how to be your own best guide. First, you need the right map to follow. Then, carefully choose the destination that is really true for you. The next step is to fully equip yourself with every quality that can assist your journey, and get rid of any excess baggage that weighs you down.

The key to success is compassion. Although the shortest distance between two points is a straight line, life often takes a zig-zag path. When it looks like you are bound in the wrong direction, don't lose heart. Instead, learn how to read the signs, enjoy the detour, and appreciate the richness that can grow from this experience. To compassionately coach yourself requires patience, consideration, willingness, courage, forgiveness, gratitude, trust and self love. Then, you perceive whatever happens as precious. You can let go of feeling driven to get somewhere. No matter where you end up, you rest happy, knowing you've enjoyed the journey.

Many people, including myself, who have used these techniques have made miraculous changes in their lives. My wish is that you can do that too. Once you become familiar with the process, you can use it again and again whenever you want to create new possibilities, opportunities and success.

Acknowledgements

Thank you to the many people who have contributed to the creation of this book:

My clients and students who have shared their experiences and taught me so much over the years, especially the people who generously gave permission to include their stories as inspiring examples.*

My friend Eileen Campbell, for her inspiration, encouragement and faith in me.

My editors Judith Kendra and Susan Lascelles, for their helpful comments that made the writing so easy.

My colleagues Charles Faulkner, Susan Martle, Jane Ferguson and Nick Owen, for their thoughtful, honest and insightful feedback, and to Wendy Harwood and Natasha Alexander for testing the exercises.

My many inspiring teachers and friends who have guided my NLP learning process: Robert Dilts, Suzi Smith, Tim Halbom, Tad James, John Overdurf, Julie Silverthorn, Julian Russell, Steve Gilligan, Robert McDonald, Tony Robbins, Ian McDermott, and Michael Neill. Plus a special mention for Duane O'Kane for awakening me with his sincere, gentle direction, support and care.

My special mentors, Chuck and Lency Spezzano, for their invaluable wisdom, compassionate insights, kind support and belief in me, and for being such great teachers of *A Course in Miracles* principles.

To the many authors and speakers who inspired me, especially Marianne Williamson, Marshall Rosenburg, Krishnamurti, Swami Anantananda and Paramahansa Yogananda.

My incredible network of friends whose love, care, support, hospitality and fun help keep my life in balance, some of whom supported me in my darkest moments, especially Brian Thorpe,

All the case studies included in this book are true stories although the names may have been altered to protect their anonymity.

Joe Powell, Sue Head, Diana MacClellan, Nicholas Pole, Ian Patrick, Steen Carndorf, Patricia Lacey and Anne Morgan.

Lastly to all the people who have asked for a book to help them learn how to open their hearts and be all they came to be.

Introduction

There is a place in you
Where there is perfect peace.
There is a place in you
Where nothing is impossible.

A Course in Miracles

Imagine you could discover the secret to creating the life of your dreams. From start to finish, this book offers easy to follow steps for learning how to coach yourself to do just that. *Compassionate Coaching* offers a banquet of different food for thought. You can graze on some of the small chunks of advice, or you can feast on the full process. Then you can learn how to put it all together. Create your own unique combination for success.

Does your life need to change? Do you know exactly what you want? Have you been puzzled about why it hasn't happened yet? Maybe you are already familiar with setting goals, and the power of positive thinking. You may also believe that anything is possible if you focus and apply enough effort. Perhaps what you keep looking for is a recipe for success. As my own quest for such a recipe began, it became obvious that some ingredients were missing.

When you coach yourself, an essential ingredient is compassion. How you motivate yourself, how you talk to yourself, how you treat yourself, and how you stand up for what is most important to you makes all the difference. How can you learn to be thankful, even when things don't turn out the way you want? How can you give yourself the best quality help and support? How can you be kind to yourself when mistakes are made? When judging and blaming stops, it is possible to choose compassion instead. Then miracles can happen.

Another key ingredient comes from storytelling. Since time began, human beings have delighted in telling stories. Gathering around campfires, performing ritual dramas, singing or play-acting tales of history and fantasy, various ways of storytelling preserved the wisdom of the ages. Often the wise elders of the tribe would pepper the ancient stories with metaphors of teaching and learning. Wandering minstrels gathered the news and travelled from village to village recounting the latest stories. Nowadays our mixture of TV soaps, musicals and movies continues this tradition.

Paramahansa Yogananda, the swami who introduced Yoga to the Western world, once described life as a 'Cosmic Motion Picture', a movie that is being projected on the screen of this earth. 'If you could see what is going on behind the screen of this life, you wouldn't suffer at all,' he said. In truth, it does seem like everyone is watching their own little life movies and taking them all very seriously. Some are dramas, some are adventures, some love stories. There are crimes of passion, triumphs over the odds, tragedies, and healing successes. Each movie, no matter how pleasant or miserable, seems precious to its owner. But what can you do if you don't like the movie you are caught up in? Who creates the movie? Is it possible to change the script? What needs to be understood, appreciated and taken into account before directing and producing a new movie?

Because thinking in stories and metaphors is so natural, using this ancient art adds surprising zest to coaching yourself. When you want to change your life, a great way to begin is to re-write your movie script. By spicing up the movies that you create in your own mind, you channel powerful unconscious energies to assist you. The trick is to make sure you choose a new script that satisfies your purpose in life, who you are, who you came to be, and who you want to become.

Some scripts don't work as well as others. You may have outlived the usefulness of an old familiar script. When you are not happy with the movie script you are living, when it doesn't match the life of your dreams, when you are reaping results you don't want, it could be a good time to re-write your script. For example, a successful artist experienced seven car accidents in seven years – all rear end collisions! This interesting metaphor raised questions about who was pushing her from behind, and creating impediments to her work. Her repetitive script had to do with competition and revenge against her father, which she was ready to change. Sometimes it takes patient detective work to discover where the problems lie, and what kind of solution will work best.

When I found myself living a trauma script, it was a definite clue that something really needed to change in my life. Having just been diagnosed with a brain tumour, I intuitively knew it wasn't only my body that needed healing. My life had been so stressful for so long, it was not surprising that my body had become ill. For years, I had known exactly what I wanted to achieve. But the more I concentrated on moving towards my positive goals, the more that emphasised how much I disliked where I was. When my life didn't improve, my unhappiness grew stronger. So I'd focus even more obsessively on achieving my positive goals! There was something wrong with this picture. It wasn't working.

No matter what I did, the results seemed disappointing. I felt discouraged. Despite this, I never gave up searching for a solution. Although I was not graced with an overnight miracle, my quest for healing helped me gain more insight and wisdom. I kept wondering what did I have to change to have my life the way I wanted it?

There must have been a problem with the way I motivated myself. Both the 'carrot' and the 'stick' approaches seemed to be working. Moving 'towards the carrot' I wanted attracted me like a magnet. Just as 'moving away from the stick' that I didn't want repelled me into action. But despite all my positive efforts, determination, and perseverance, not only did my goals elude me, but I ended up frustrated and confused. In an effort to find out what was wrong, I started looking into the metaphors and deeper stories behind my script.

My fascination with stories and metaphor began when I was working as an artist. It was obvious that not only does the visual image have multiple meanings, but each colour carries different feelings, and every brush stroke reveals different emotions. Every little detail carries meaning. The way people dress – no matter how conventionally or unconventionally – is their costume. If you look closely enough, their clothes, jewellery, grooming, posture, gestures and facial expression, can tell you what kind of role they are acting out in their own script. Everything tells a story.

The more you find out about a person: how they live, how they decorate their homes, how they do what they do; the more about their life scripts you will discover. Each person travels through their own personal landscape of life to find their path. Their demeanour, their attitude, will give you clues as to how much they have enjoyed the journey so far.

My appreciation of life scripts grew during my career in Mind/Body medicine, working as a naturopath and osteopath. I became fascinated with the metaphors of the body. When a person had a stiff, painful neck, there was often a story about someone being a 'pain in the neck' for them. When they couldn't walk, there was usually a situation where they did not want to move forward, or steps they didn't want to take. As more patients came to me, there always seemed to be a direct correlation between their physical symptoms and the problems in their lives. It was impossible not to notice that health problems often directly reflected life problems. I began to wonder what would happen if you dealt with the life script problems. Would the health problems disappear?

One day I had an unforgettable session with a young woman with eczema that convinced me that this was more than mere coincidence. This particular twenty-year-old had come to see me with lower back problems, but she mentioned that she had very bad eczema on her hands that might be due to some allergy. After treating her back, I looked at her hands, which were both red, swollen, and covered with flaking skin and deep cracks which were bleeding slightly. They looked extremely painful and angry. We decided to 'talk' to the imaginary part of her that was creating the eczema to find out what it was about. The hands are about doing, touching and caring. Her eczema looked like a snake trying to shed its skin, and it also made the purpose of her hands impossible. What could she be longing to do or to touch, that created so much anger and frustration?

The life script she was living concerned her parents, who had been going through an ugly separation and divorce. Being the only child, she often felt torn between the two of them, right in the middle of all the stress and tugs of war. This part of her just wanted all the fighting to stop. She wanted a happy home. She wanted peace. Suddenly she realised that her eczema-covered hands were expressing all the anger she felt inside – even though she was acting sweet and nice. She then decided what was true for her: to choose peace, rather than to hold on to being angry.

She was already very spiritually orientated, so she knew how to get in touch with her own inner peaceful state of mind. So I invited her to do so, as an antidote to all the stress she had been experiencing. Only thirty minutes had passed as we chatted, so when we happened to look back at her hands, we were both astonished to see both hands looking absolutely perfect. There was no trace of redness, swelling, cracks or flakes. The eczema had completely disappeared. Her mother, who had been sitting a few feet away, was in stunned silence throughout the process. Astounded, she told us that she had watched the transformation take place while we had been chatting.

As is the human body, so is the cosmic body.
As is the human mind, so is the cosmic mind.
As is the microcosm, so is the macrocosm.

Ayurvedic saying

My curiosity about the stories we write with our lives became a serious exploration when I was first diagnosed with a small and inoperable brain tumour. What a shock! It felt like the cancer had come out of nowhere and had nothing to do with me. I felt helpless. There was no safe place to run to. Suddenly my own body felt like a war zone, invaded by unfriendly cells that were acting undercover. I couldn't see or feel or touch my tumour. It was only detectable by MRI scans and blood tests. The threat of possibly having to endure surgery, radiation and chemotherapy was terrifying.

For years, I had been puzzled about the cause of the intense headaches I suffered much too often. Now I knew there was a physical reason for them, but I had to wonder if my headaches were also a message. I began to wonder if this tumour had a purpose.

All my life, my dream script had been to get married and

have a happy family. I had married, but my husband didn't want children. After we grew apart and later got divorced, my dream script became all about finding my perfect partner, getting re-married and having children. It didn't seem too much to ask. Curiously, what I didn't know was that the side effect of my brain tumour was infertility, due to the excess hormones produced. The irony of my situation could not be overlooked.

Rather than just thinking my tumour was bad luck, I began to wonder if there was another script running outside of my conscious awareness . . . and so began my adventurous exploration into the hidden realms of my own mind, metaphors and life scripts.

At first, no one could tell if my tumour was benign or malignant. After many tests, scans and examinations, and after thoroughly researching the few medical solutions possible, I chose not to take the drugs or surgery. Instead, with the support of my specialist, an enlightened endocrinologist, I chose to experiment with alternative methods. Intuitively, I felt that my tumour was the direct result of stress. For nearly ten years my life had been an emotional roller coaster ride of relationship disasters. The more I moved towards fulfilling my happy family dream, the more impossible situations developed. Something was wrong.

Because my tumour was so deeply hidden, sometimes it didn't feel real. It was easy to believe I could heal a cold, or a cut finger, but something as complicated as cancer felt off-the-scale impossible. One of the first 'turnarounds' in my thinking however, was when a friend suggested that I visualise my tumour as being the same as a cut finger. Just as I could trust that my body could heal a small cut, I could trust that my body could rectify these aberrant cells. After all, if my body had created this tumour, it knew exactly how to un-create it.

There is no order of difficulty in miracles. One is not harder or bigger than another. They are all the same. All expressions of love are maximal.

A Course in Miracles

Not knowing what had caused this cancer to appear, how could I know what would help to heal it? Even more troubling, there was no way of knowing whether it would get worse or not. In fact, it did get a lot worse at first, and my specialists increased their pressure on me to take the suppressive drugs. The stress of maintaining my course despite lack of improvements was almost more stressful than having the tumour.

Every thought you think and every feeling you feel releases different chemical messengers into your body. These hormones either rejuvenate and relax your body or cause tension, wear and tear. Your mind and heart therefore affect your physical body every moment. Therefore, your habitual thoughts and feelings indirectly create either health or ill health.

Your thoughts and feelings are also connected to your perception. According to research, over two million bits of information bombard your senses every second. Out of that, your brain receives only seven, plus or minus two, bits of information per second. Your habitual ways of thinking literally filter out the rest. So you see, hear, and feel only what you choose. If you change your thinking, then your perception of a situation will also change.

Your mind doesn't realise that your perception deleted millions of bits of information. It believes your perceived problems are real and urges you to do something. When you don't know what to do though, your mind cleverly hides the problem, sometimes allowing you to forget all about it. Often these hidden thoughts and beliefs continue to create the most troublesome 'realities' you have to deal with. By re-writing the script of your life, you can gently direct your perception of reality to see what is true.

Everything that happens is an opportunity for healing your life. When I was healing my brain tumour, my first mistake was to believe that the aberrant cells were the problem. On the physical level, an illness – whether it is cancer, or a cold – seems to be a collection of bodily symptoms. On a deeper level, the problem must be the habitual thoughts and feelings that led to the creation of the illness. If you focus on only the physical symptoms of a disease, you may not find a complete solution. What is needed is a change of perception. When the mind is healed and at peace, then the physical problem no longer has a purpose. Then the path to healing is easy.

Of course, when my regular scans showed no change at all, those tumour cells seemed pretty convincing and real. However, once again, it was a wise friend who pointed out that although 'something' was showing on the scans *at the moment the scan was done*, I couldn't be sure what was going on in those extra cells, or how fast they might heal. They might be empty scar tissue, or they might be healing right this moment. They may have healed already, after the scan was done.

Could everything be related to your thoughts? Clearly, you see reality according to your beliefs and perception. That is why no two people observe exactly the same event. But this is good news, because it means that by learning how to change your thoughts, beliefs and perception, you can change much more. The universe does not write your scripts or cause things to happen to you without your input and participation. You have the freedom to creatively respond to whatever life offers. You can learn from life by looking at things differently. If you could monitor your thoughts more carefully and become more aware, if you could let go of your scripts long enough to be still, perhaps you could hear what you need to know, and act from a place of inner peace.

On a superficial level, I felt that my brain tumour was the most unfair thing that could have happened to me. All I had ever wanted was to have a loving relationship, with healthy children – a happy family. My tumour not only invaded my relationship but also caused infertility. Even I couldn't miss this strange co-incidence! Looking deeper, I slowly discovered many old wounds that required gentle unravelling and resolution. Issues to do with heartbreaks, fear of sacrifice, fear of commitment, and fear of being a mother. It took a long time to finally realise that I was so full of hidden layers of fear that in fact, the last thing in the world I really wanted was a relationship with children! No wonder my body had created a tumour so perfectly designed to do as I had (unconsciously) asked.

Miracles are natural. When they do not occur, something has gone wrong.

A Course in Miracles

Whilst seeking different ways to balance the physical aspects of the tumour, I began to study NLP (Neuro-Linguistic Programming) and various forms of practical psychology, as well as every book I could find on healing relationship problems. Clinical psychologist, Dr Chuck Spezzano and his wife Lency Spezzano inspired me so much with their specialist work on relationships that I became one of their advanced trainers and studied with them for ten years.

The techniques of NLP helped tremendously to calm down my stress levels. Through various different processes and exercises, I was able to heal many of my early life experiences, feelings and decisions that had contributed to creating my tumour. Gradually, after a few years, the hormone production of my tumour decreased to a stable, but still too high, level. My specialist was surprised though, and began encouraging me to keep doing whatever it was I was doing. Because the tumour was now stable, he also decided that it was benign.

I used to think that if I did everything 'right', then my tumour would disappear. But what I didn't realise was that my intense desire to make it go away, was actually investing in making my tumour real. It was my old obsession with focusing on getting my goal again! This attachment to getting some kind of outcome, or getting needs met is very confusing. Many people focus on goals, whether it is getting rich or having a perfect relationship or solving some problem, and think if everything is done right, it will magically happen. But this is a trap! If it doesn't happen the way you want it, you can feel like a failure.

Investing your energy in external factors, in order to find happiness doesn't work. You would be wiser to invest in your peace of mind. The solution that heals comes with the miracle of forgiveness, love and joining with others. When you invest in your peace of mind, when you are willing to see yourself as innocent, when you forgive others, the doors to healing and success open. The abundance of the universe can then deliver whatever you want that is appropriate.

When I first realised that focusing on being well wasn't helping, I really didn't know what to do instead. How do you not focus on what you want? How could I stop thinking about what was obsessing me? One of my first teachers, Krishnamurti, once wrote that if you want to make something holy, put the object on your mantelpiece, and worship it everyday. Bring it flowers, light a candle, put incense around it, chant some mantras and it will soon become holy for you, not because there is any inherent holiness in it, but merely because you have given it that holiness by believing it to be holy. Even though wanting to be well is a perfectly natural and good intention, I realised I had turned it into an obsession.

Whenever you invest your mind like this in a particular solution, especially if you become attached to some outcome or result, you make that more important than your unlimited potential. Being too attached to an outcome limits you and can possibly prevent an even bigger outcome from happening. You may have this mantelpiece in your mind on an unconscious level without realising it. You may not even know that you have these attachments. When I finally let go of needing my tumour to disappear, when I finally accepted that it would probably be with me to the end of my days, when I truly regarded it as my friend and teacher, when I felt gratitude for the motivation it had given me to change my life and my thinking, when I had forgiven all the people I had grudges with, its presence in my body didn't bother me anymore.

It may surprise you, but every problem you have, everywhere you are not at peace, can be traced to a lack of forgiveness. Check this out for yourself: think of a problem you have and notice whom you could be holding a grudge against (sometimes it is yourself, or fate). Often these grudges began long, long ago, before you had the ability to understand or view things from a better perspective. The old wounds got forgotten, covered up, and buried deep, hidden from your conscious awareness. They may be rumbling under the surface of your behaviour. Have you ever over-reacted with a sense of 'justifiable' rage or feelings of revenge? You forget that these grudges may be based on a mistaken perception of events. The old scripts written so long ago, feel like the truth. Back then, it could have seemed like a fight for survival. You may have felt all alone, separate and frightened that your needs would not be met. The universe probably felt like a frightening place where you were vulnerable and small. How could you have known there are other ways to think?

What truly heals is remembering that you are a vital part of this vast miraculous universe and you are not alone. You need to move away from problem solving long enough to be able to monitor your thoughts. You need to let go of your needs long enough to be still, and listen. You need to turn within and ask for help and inner guidance. You need to forgive. You cannot create miracles if you believe you are alone.

While seeking to heal my tumour, I continued to study and work through my personal issues for several years, gradually accumulating certificates and diplomas in several different fields. My career changed as I began to share what I had learned. It slowly dawned on me that my tumour had actually been a great motivator. Without it, I probably would not have been so dedicated or persistent in my studies. After ten years, instead of being frustrated by what seemed to be a lack of healing, I began to appreciate that my tumour must still have some positive purpose for me. Since it had done such a good job directing me to study and grow in so many ways, it made sense to trust whatever reason it might have for staying with me. Maybe it was keeping me humble! Perhaps it was just making sure that I would persist in learning ways to keep my life, my thoughts and my feelings in balance. Maybe it had a bigger script for my life.

I will never forget the day I walked into my doctor's office with my annual blood test results. The lab report showed that the hormone levels were well within the normal range. Probably because I had fully accepted the presence of the tumour, I thought the result must be a mistake, even though my headaches had diminished as well. So when my doctor took one look at the results and said, 'Wow! That's amazing!' I was surprised. When I questioned him, he insisted that it could only mean that my tumour had regressed to normal. He said, 'I don't know how you have done this, but it is a real credit to you. I've been seeing you every year, and watched you change. You are not the same person I met ten years ago.' It was a poignant moment, because although I had never taken any of the medication he prescribed, his monitoring had been vital throughout my journey. As I appreciated his support, I realised what an important part he had played. In fact, so many people had helped me on my journey, I began to think of them all as my team.

Throughout my journey of discovery, I've enjoyed sharing what I've learned with my private clients as well as teaching these skills in my classes. Although this path may not be easy, it has helped many people to achieve astonishing results. Now I'd like to share, through this book, the processes that help to produce miraculous change. Re-writing the script of your life can help you get a whole new perspective on your life. Doing the simple exercises, will help you to find solutions to particular problems you might have. You can get back on track and be more aligned with who you have come to be, living your true purpose. The processes will work best when you follow the exercises as you read through each chapter.

The book has been carefully designed to help you reconnect with your inner resources and assist you to make whatever changes you want. It is not meant to be a substitute for proper medical treatment. Nor is it intended to replace the need for thorough training if you are intending to work with clients. What it can do is give you a framework that helps you put your inner wisdom into action.

Thanks to my tumour, my life took a very different path, and I am happy with the person I have become. I feel more akin to my purpose than ever before and more able to share my talents and give my gifts. I believe that like snowflakes, everyone is unique. Everyone holds a special place in the complete hologram of the universe. The world simply would not be complete without each person performing their unique role and function. Each person has special gifts they bring into this world, talents to share, potential for change and personal evolution. Each life has a purpose, maybe several purposes.

Sometimes you can get embroiled in your old miserable scripts and forget who you came here to be. You forget your purpose. You forget who you really are. You keep yourself too small and limit the scope of your life. You forget how connected you are to the unlimited potential. This book invites you to remember again.

Dare to Dream

All people dream, but not all equally. Those who dream by night in the dusty recesses of their minds wake in the day to find it was vanity; but the dreamers of the day are dangerous, for they may act their dreams with open eyes, to make it possible.

LAWRENCE OF ARABIA

Have you ever wished you could create a Dream Script of how you would like your life to be? Maybe you have contemplated a whole new career, but feel unsure about taking such a different direction? Perhaps you've wanted to change something about your relationship? Or you might have a fitness or health issue that needs healing? If only there was a magic wand that could whisk away all the difficulties and make miracles happen! Throughout my own healing journey, I searched for just such a magic pathway. I urgently needed to find what really works. What helps miraculous change and healing take place? This question guided my quest: to create a map for coaching people to manifest their dreams.

After years of research, exploring and integrating many different techniques, I noticed there was a basic structure of thinking that seemed to help people. When my clients began to reap wonderful results, I was encouraged. When my students were able to learn and use the same techniques successfully, I gained confidence. When my own healing crisis resolved, I was convinced. The pattern that had emerged from working with thousands of clients consistently produced great changes. But could anyone learn this pattern and structure and use it with ease?

I've designed this book carefully to deliver both the structure of thinking and some of the essential patterns of behaviour that produce results in coaching. You can gain useful insights just through reading the stories in each chapter, and understanding the inner journeys of each client. By following the exercises diligently as well, you can have fun learning the complete process for yourself. Are you curious enough to test the process out for yourself to see if it works? Wouldn't it be amazing if you started manifesting the life of your dreams?

Designing a Dream Script for Your Life

What if you could design a Dream Script for the rest of your life and channel your mind to achieve it? What would you like to have happen? Where would you be, what would you be doing, what kind of people would you be with? What would you be learning, how would you be developing and growing? How would you be giving and sharing yourself? Who would you be? What would you believe is possible? What if you could learn a pattern of thinking that would help you to achieve all your dreams? Here in this book, you can discover the secrets of how to make positive changes that really work.

How long has it been since you asked yourself what you really want in life? Maybe you never have! If you are like most people, you have vague ideas about how you would like your life to be, but you don't spend much time thinking about it. Perhaps you may even believe that doing so would be nothing more than unrealistic daydreams or wishful thinking that serve no purpose. But not tapping into your imagination, not using your lateral thinking brain, means that you waste more than ninety per cent of your creative energy. Are you aware that everything ever created by man began by someone dreaming it first? When your imaginative power is engaged, you can achieve what seems impossible. Now you can learn how to do this by following simple exercises that work with this creative part of your mind.

Nothing happens unless first a dream.

Carl Sandburg

What you might not realise is that whether you think you are following your dreams or not, part of your mind is running stories about who you are, what you are capable of, how well you do what you do, what kind of success and relationships you deserve, and even how fit or unfit you can be. These scripts are already programming your behaviour and the results you get. When they bring you success you probably feel happy. But when things go wrong, you would be wise to wonder about the programmes that have been installed. It might be smart to learn how to update them. Where did these stories come from?

If you think of your brain as a computer, you are born with a basic hard drive. Then as you grow up, parents, carers, teachers, friends and colleagues start installing software. All the events of your life, everything that happens, as well as how you feel about everything, gets recorded and stored as data. If you are not getting the results you would like in life, begin to suspect that there is a glitch in your software, or that the information stored has not been processed properly or filed appropriately. There may even be a computer virus running amok! Many people's minds are all jumbled up and confused like a computer gone haywire. It is no surprise that what comes out is random actions and stupid behaviours! Wouldn't it make more sense to sort out what programmes are running? Don't you think that if you could train your mind, you could learn how to channel your energy for better results? Unlike computers, you can learn ways to mend even the most corrupted programmes. You don't have to believe that what your life has been like so far is who you are. The past does not have to equal the future.

Some coaching practices advise working towards small attainable goals, so as to avoid disappointment. Whilst this is very safe and easy to measure, it doesn't activate the dynamic part of your creative mind. It simply isn't exciting enough! Limiting yourself to little goals may or may not help you make the radical changes you might really want. If you need to make big changes, you need to be totally honest and in alignment with your innermost desires. If you limit yourself to little goals, tiny changes that you know are attainable, you might be thinking too small. Dare to believe you could have what you really want, and ask yourself questions like this:

- If you could be sure of success, what would you choose?
- If you knew you couldn't fail, what would you dare to do?
- If you were sure you could be happy, what would you change?

Lots of people get so involved with the day-to-day running of their lives that they just forget how creative their minds can be. Our brains are much more sophisticated and complex than any computer ever invented. There are untapped energies in your unconscious mind that can help you do whatever you want and have whatever is true for you. How do you tap into this powerful source? By learning how to work with your mind compassionately and playfully, you can start to manifest your dreams into reality. These parts of your mind think in stories, dreams and metaphors, so it is important to speak this kind of language so that your unconscious mind listens. This book deliberately uses many stories of what worked for other people in order to appeal to the story-loving part of your mind. Each story shares different secrets of how to access your unconscious mind. Just follow the exercises throughout the book to discover what programmes are already running in your mind. Then you can make the necessary adjustments so that you can manifest the changes you really want.

The suggestions and exercises throughout this book are carefully designed to help you be thorough and safe throughout your exploration, step by step. The complete structure will reveal the process of how to make your dreams come true. You can also learn how to help others achieve their dreams. By following the steps carefully, you can re-discover what your dreams are, what gifts you have come to give, and what your purpose is. Along the way, it will also be important to assess what hidden needs might need to be recognised and be dealt with, and to work through any issues that might be holding you back. When you have thoroughly cleared the path to your dreams, the last chapter will teach you how to harness the energies to make your dreams a reality.

If there is only one particular area of your life that needs improvement, you can direct all the exercises throughout the book to help you achieve a specific result. You can also achieve major breakthroughs in several different areas all at once, but you may need to repeat some of the exercises to address each different goal. Both approaches work well.

I believe that the very purpose of our life is to seek happiness. That is clear. Whether one believes in religion or not, whether one believes in this religion or that religion, we all are seeking something better in life. So, I think, the very motion of our life is towards happiness . . . I believe that happiness can be achieved through training the mind.

H. H. Dalai Lama

Ask most people what they want, and they invariably say 'I want to be happy'. But what they believe will bring them happiness can vary a lot. Some people think achieving great success and abundance will bring happiness. Some believe it requires having perfect relationships and great sex. Some think being able to buy all the best toys, clothes, expensive homes and holidays will bring them happiness. Some would be happy if they could just be healthy and fit. Some want to be creative artists or musicians. Some believe only spiritual enlightenment can bring true happiness. And then there are some that don't even know what would make them happy! Most people spend their lives trying to achieve whatever they believe will bring them happiness. But they haven't bothered to find out if their plan for happiness will deliver what they want!

Strangely enough, whenever I ask groups to visualise their happiest dream, at least half the room find it completely impossible. They can't imagine a positive script for their lives. The idea does not compute. They don't know what they want – although some of them can go on for hours about what they don't want! Even though people complain about their lives, they often don't have any idea what they would like instead. Sometimes they are so attached to their current script being real, the exercise seems like a pointless fantasy. Maybe they don't believe they deserve to have what they want. Could it be that NOT knowing what you want is a major factor of you not having the life of your dreams? If you can, at least focus on some specific goals you would be willing to put in your script. If you can imagine a few wonderful things happening in specific areas of your life, you are making a good start.

If you can't imagine what you would put in the Dream Script of your life, think about all the things you love to do in your life right now, no matter how frivolous. Notice what kind of books and magazines you love to read, what kind of movies excite you, what activities you feel enthusiastic about, what you enjoy best when you have free time. Imagine you could video yourself throughout each day . . . what interests and fascinates you? If you make a list of all your favourite activities and interests, it will give you valuable clues about what should be included in your Dream Script. Make a list:

- All the activities you love best to do.
- What books and magazines you read avidly.
- What kind of movies you enjoy.
- Your hobbies, sports, leisure activities.
- Whatever you find fun, exciting, fascinating.

....

If the idea of imagining a Dream Script for your life completely turns you off, or you can't do it for some other reason, you can start at the middle of the book and work through the exercises in Chapters 4, 5, and 6, before you come back to do Chapters 1, 2, and 3. Then you'll be ready to manifest your dreams coming true in Chapters 7 and 8.

....

Being Happy

Most people say that they just want to be happy and they just want happiness for others too. That's great. Happiness is a true state of mind that you can have anywhere, anytime. But just for fun, get in touch with the ideas, dreams and fantasies you might have for what would bring you that happiness. Don't worry about how it will happen, or what could get in the way. Resist editing the positive ideas that come into your mind. Dream your dream of how you would like your life to be.

You want to be happy.
You want peace.
You do not have them now,
Because your mind is totally undisciplined.

A Course in Miracles

Getting an idea of what you would like to have in your Dream Script is only the first step. Each chapter in the book will take you through different processes to help you set the scene for your Script to become a reality. Sometimes the hardest part is knowing what you want. There are many pitfalls that can get in the way. You can learn from the stories and experience of others to make your journey much easier. Remember, the part of your mind that you most need to get to know and under-stand – your subconscious mind – listens and learns best through stories and metaphors. So, throughout this book, just relax and keep your mind open, as you read about other people's stories – like the one that follows.

Mary was a great example of someone who always thought she knew exactly what she wanted, and her life seemed full of results that proved it! As an IT Sales Director in her thirties, she lived what appeared to be a highly successful life, despite a difficult childhood and two failed marriages. Then she became very ill with glandular fever, from which she never seemed to fully recover. Had it developed into M.E. or was she just burnt out? She became so deeply depressed that her doctor wanted to admit her to hospital. She agreed to take Prozac instead, but was still put under psychiatric supervision for six months. In fact, depression was nothing new for her. She admitted that she had suffered bouts of depression since she was fifteen, due to family problems and splitting up with her first boyfriend.

Her doctor told her that her depression was hereditary and there was nothing she could do about it. She would always have to take Prozac. But she just wouldn't accept that. Somewhere deep inside, she felt that this was just not who she was meant to be. Later, her problems were labelled as M.E. but she felt she was just being given excuses. She couldn't accept that her life could only be happy if she took a pill. She became deter-mined to find another way.

After two years of low energy, she came off the Prozac and started having serious attacks of depression. Sometimes she would hit rock bottom for days and then stay low for weeks. But she was good at hiding it, somehow finding ways to cope, and still managing to hold down her stressful job! Some days she thought she would crash. Most people thought she was a highly-strung, hard-nosed businesswoman. Then after another relationship broke up, she suffered a really bad bout of depression. Persistently continuing her search for a way through her problems, she attended one of my training seminars where I was teaching the *Compassionate Coaching* methods.

After seeing counsellors for fifteen years, she was fed up with being told 'to love yourself, be kind to yourself and love your inner child'. She said if one more person told her that, she'd hit them! If she knew how to do that, she wouldn't be there getting counselling! Through learning *Compassionate Coaching* techniques with me she finally developed an understanding of her own unconscious mind, that inner child that needed her love. Finally, she had an idea of how to have a relationship with a part of herself she had never known before.

Although she had been so exhausted by the M.E. that she hardly had any energy to think about changing her life script, she was so inspired by what she learned from *Compassionate Coaching*, that she decided to work towards changing her career completely and become a trainer herself. During one exercise, she suddenly imagined an exciting picture of herself as a trainer, and working with children. She remembered that she had always felt drawn to working with children. She began to dream a whole new ideal life script.

Learning the techniques in this book gave her the tools she needed to make sense of her whole life. She imagined using a remote control whenever she didn't like the movies she was running in her mind – she'd just change the channel! It was great to feel she had more choice. Unfortunately, her habitual thinking habits had been running for so many years, that despite all the new tools, her health wasn't getting any better. She became angry and impatient with this lack of progress. She still suffered bouts of depression despite having worked through many layers of old beliefs. It felt like a never ending black hole, and her old pessimism dragged her down again.

Finally a big turning point came during a coaching session, when she faced her blackest, most depressing, thoughts and realised that she was blaming God for all her problems. It felt like she had done something wrong, and that an angry God was punishing her – hence she now hated God! She intuitively sensed that this had all started when she was in the womb. Something was not right back then, and she sensed her mother was angry with her as a baby in the womb. Not being able to understand what was going on, she decided she must have done something really bad. (Later on, her mother revealed that she hadn't been married during her pregnancy and this had caused a great deal of stress.) With the wisdom of hindsight, she was gradually able to see the innocence of that little baby in the womb. She realised that God wasn't punishing her. She healed her anger towards God, and began to feel comfortable being a small part of something really big.

Deciding to make changes in her life, she quit her job, leaving behind the fifteen-year IT career that she had worked so hard at building up. Surprisingly she felt nothing but relief, even though she had no new job to take its place. Suddenly she was home alone, without her income, without her sports car, and no longer the successful, super efficient, independent, businesswoman. She no longer had an identity. If she wasn't that IT Sales Director, who was she? She got scared and felt quite lost. But she kept continuing with her studies and gradually achieved all the qualifications to be a trainer. Despite some tough setbacks when her beloved grandmother died, despite still battling with some lingering symptoms of M.E., and despite bits of her old self-hatred re-surfacing from time to time, she continued to use the *Compassionate Coaching* skills to help get her out of the holes.

Finally, only eighteen months after she dreamt up her new life script, she began to feel something had shifted. She noticed that she was feeling physically better and more empowered. She realised that whatever she wanted, seemed to be manifesting in her life, often without any effort on her part. She laughingly told me that she had bought a second-hand car that she loathed and wanted to get rid of. While it was parked outside her house, someone drove right into it and smashed it beyond repair. With her insurance payment, she replaced it with a car she liked! Then, to solve her money problems, she received £5000 as a surprise gift when she needed it most. A few days later, she could hardly believe it when she was offered jobs both as a trainer and working with children! This meant she could maintain her income without working a punishing schedule and without having to use her old pushy sales strategies. Instead, she now found that she was able to attract whatever she wanted.

On her recent check-up, her doctor said he had never seen her look so healthy. So encouraged by her successes, she began to believe even more confidently that she could manifest the life of her dreams. Over lunch with a friend, she shared that she was finally ready to risk having a new relationship. The next day, her friend called and invited her to a party where she met a wonderful man and fell in love. He shared her dream of moving to Spain and now they are in the process of creating a centre there. All this happened so quickly and easily, it was almost unbeliveable. Maybe dreams can come true.

Your imagination is your preview of life's coming attractions.
Albert Einstein

Raising Your Awareness: what results are you getting?

Many people believe that they are already doing everything they can to create happiness. How much effort do you put in every day to make things happen to bring you some form of satisfaction and happiness? You may find that your efforts are rewarded, and lots of happy events unfold. Perhaps you might be forced to notice, however, that despite your good efforts, everything seems to go wrong, and you don't end up happy. If you are like many people, you might have been tempted to blame other people or bad luck or whatever, rather than do a re-assessment of your original efforts.

Quickly think of a number between 1 and 10 for each of the following questions:

- How happy are you?
- How much effort are you making right now to create more happiness?
- If you can be objective, how successful have you been, so far? How well did you score?

With the best of intentions, and wanting everyone to be happy, some people can be amazingly blind about the results they are getting. They keep on doing what makes sense for them, thinking that everyone else will appreciate what they are doing. Or if they notice that what they are doing isn't working, they just blame everyone else for creating problems. They think there is something wrong with the other people for not thinking the way they do or for not behaving appropriately.

If you find yourself stuck in situations where no matter what you say or do, you never seem to get the responses you want, begin to suspect that some of your old programming needs updating. If what you are doing isn't working, it is time to learn something new. There is a useful principle from NLP (Neuro Linguistic Programming) that states: 'The meaning of the communication is the response you get.' This means that when you say something, other people may not hear it the way you mean it. Your listener may interpret your message quite differently and react to the meaning they make of it, rather than what you intended. If you want them to understand your meaning, then you must keep changing the way that you communicate that message until their understanding matches your meaning. This can require lots of patience and understanding. Just because you may think that you say things very clearly does not guarantee that other people listen and hear things as clearly.

Words are not exact; each word you use is actually a symbol or metaphor. Some words have such complex meanings, or multiple meanings, that it becomes easy to misunderstand what is said. Different people attach different meanings to words and the way that they are said. The following story illustrates how it is possible to raise your awareness, notice when you are not getting the results you want, and make the necessary adjustments.

Unhappy Results

A mother of three teenagers was at her wits end. She felt lonely, exhausted, guilty and under attack. Despite being married for twenty-two years, she was threatening divorce since the last ten years had been so very unhappy. Her husband had also taken to drinking excessively. 'No matter what I say or do to support him, he feels criticised,' she said. 'He just has this negative attitude and says there's no point in talking to me.'

Her three children were all equally challenging in different ways: one was rebellious, smoking, drinking and having problems at school; one was suffering from being bullied and abused; and the third was refusing to take necessary medications for a health problem. All three complained about how she was always nagging them. The atmosphere at home was miserable. Then her in-laws remarked how unkind, sharp and unfriendly she was. When they found out that she was threatening to leave her husband, they viciously told her how they had never liked her from day one!

Despite this feedback from her family, this woman persisted in believing that she was giving nothing but love to her family, and doing everything she could to make everyone happy! In fact, she reported somewhat righteously how she had taken on over-time in order to fund improvements for their home. In addition, her intention behind all the 'good advice' she gave everyone was to create the perfect scene for happiness. But something was very wrong with this picture! Despite all the effort she put into trying to get her husband and children to behave properly, no one was happy – least of all her!

I asked her for some examples of the good advice she gave to her family, and it soon became clear that she had some very specific expectations of how everyone should behave at all times. It was crucial for her to be considered a good mother and a good wife, and she couldn't understand why no one appreciated her directives. She had become a tyrant, shouting louder and louder when none of them appeared to listen or do what they were told. Her rigid rules were making everyone's life a misery.

We talked about how much easier it would be to get her loved ones on her side if she used kindness instead of demands. What if she praised them instead of criticising? What if she gave them unconditional love instead of pouncing on every mistake and misdemeanour? Maybe that would create the loving atmosphere she so longed for. We talked about her importance as a role model in the family, being the fountain of unconditional love and nurturing. We discussed specific ways she could communicate better with her children, avoiding evaluations and judgements.

But she persisted in complaining about her husband and judging him negatively for being so depressed. I asked her what would it be like if he was the complete opposite: What if he was 'happy, happy, happy' all the time? Suddenly she started crying as she realised that then he wouldn't NEED her anymore. She had created the situation of her family being so difficult so that she could be needed by them all. It was an old script from her childhood being replayed all over again.

When she was seven years old, her youngest brother was born, and since her parents worked very hard in their bakery, she was given the job of looking after the children, which she did to perfection. She was such a natural carer, she even appointed herself as advisor to her mother. However, she was surprised when her mother did not follow her advice to divorce her father when he went on a drinking binge (he did this only once a year). She took a hard line on most things, always trying too hard to make everything perfect. Throughout her school days, she impressed everyone with how responsibly and well she behaved. And so the attitude of trying too hard had become quite a habit.

Could she let go of this? Of course, it was possible. But she was most hard on herself, and most judgemental about her own inadequacies. So the unconditional love had to begin with forgiving herself for making mistakes, and allowing others to be less than perfect too. Because she really wanted her family to be happy though, she totally committed herself to making these changes. In only one week, she made significant progress with her husband, improving their communication and restoring their relationship. Her eldest son noticed the difference in her behaviour immediately. She had stopped shouting and criticising. Now she continues to practise new ways of understanding, appreciating and encouraging her children without nagging, criticising or judging.

That which we persist in doing becomes easier – not that the nature of the task has changed, but an ability to do it has increased.

Ralph Waldo Emerson

Learning how to be observant about your communication is a skill you can develop. Many people have misconceptions about how other people perceive what they say and do. If you are not sure, ask your close friends for feedback. When you don't get the responses you expect from people, find out why. They might be receiving very different messages than the ones you thought you were sending. The sooner you correct mistakes like this, the better your communication will become. The responses you receive will also give you honest feedback about where you could improve.

Non-verbal Communication

It is important to understand that communication is not only verbal, but also has non-verbal elements such as voice tone, gestures, posture, attitude, even the way you dress. In fact, everything you do, your whole way of being is a metaphorical communication. When you walk into a room, everyone experiences you, your energy and your whole persona. Complete strangers will accurately assess each other in seconds, reading these unconscious communications. Friends and relatives are able to tell exactly what mood you are in by how you say 'Hello' when picking up the phone. It is unavoidable, so it pays to put some attention into what unconscious communications you might be giving wherever you go.

Being Too Specific Too Soon

Your Dream Script needs to stay on the dream level until you have carefully assessed whether or not all the goals it includes will really bring you happiness or not. It helps to be flexible and free of demands. Instead of being overly prescriptive about exactly what will bring you happiness, allow there to be some leeway. Aim for the happiness, but be less concerned with exactly how it is delivered.

A trap some people fall into happens when they get too attached to having life be a certain way, or about being with a certain person. Supposing you needed some form of transportation to get you somewhere and you decided you wanted a bicycle, when in fact, the universe wanted to send you a beautiful new car! You might limit your possibilities if you are overly specific in your thinking. The ideal Dream Script is one where you stretch your limits to think as big as you can. Really dare to reach for the stars and choose what really makes your heart sing! But also notice that it could arrive in different colours. It might not look exactly like what you have pictured in your imagination. Your ideal Dream Script guidelines are:

- Think big!
- Be flexible about the details.
- Avoid being too specific about certain people, places or things.

The world is full of evidence that shows the recipe for success begins with working hard for something, and staying determined to keep going for it no matter what happens. Persistence pays off. Many people make things happen through hard work, discipline, practice and control. Teachers in many professions consider these very desirable qualities. But sometimes, when those qualities are applied too early to the wrong goal, it can end in misery. It is possible to overdo discipline. Over control can become a habit. You can have too much of a good thing! When you demand so much of yourself that you become your own tyrant, where do kindness and self-love come in? This unusual tale reveals a surprising solution.

Too Much of a Good Thing

A very pretty, petite young woman with orange-striped hair and vixen eyes came to see me about her constant, incurable headaches. Something about her manner reminded me of fairies – she looked so like a pixie. She smiled strangely as she told me how she had suffered these headaches for over ten years and that no one had been able to help her. Even as we spoke, she had intense pain in her head.

When she was seven, she decided she wanted to be a gymnast and underwent intensive training with a rather cruel national coach until she was eleven. He cursed and criticised her constantly, making her focus harder and harder to perfect her mistakes.

Then she discovered ballet. She loved ballet so much she talked her father into letting her leave school to train professionally. Ballet school was gruelling and she had no friends or social life. Her life became an endless routine of trying to reach perfection. At the age of thirteen, she began suffering such bad headaches, that she found it difficult to continue her ballet training.

Years followed of all kinds of therapy: brain scans, medical drugs, teeth extractions, even an operation on her jaw. Then she started taking recreational drugs to escape the pain. She became addicted to Ecstasy and heroin. Later she was put in hospital for psychiatric help. When medicinal drugs didn't work, she began to try different forms of alternative medicine. During this time, she gave up ballet completely and tried to take up contemporary dance instead, but couldn't do much because the constant headaches were too painful.

It seemed to her as though her headaches were almost a form of punishment, but she didn't have any obvious source of guilt. However, when she started talking about her father and what a close relationship they had, her headache suddenly became so intense and unbearable, she thought her head was about to explode.

We created an imaginary energy circuit – a pathway down her arm – to drain the pain away until she was comfortable again. She described her headache as a huge black jagged 'rock' bigger than her head. Talking to the 'rock', it became clear that the 'rock's' main issue was about feeling 'not good enough'. This familiar belief was so strong that she had given up trying years ago. The headaches – which had completely stopped her from doing anything – actually served the purpose of sparing her the embarrassment of everyone finding out that she was not good enough. But of course, the disadvantage was that she couldn't do what she loved best: dance!

Unable to ignore the subconscious metaphors of her hair, dress and eyes, I decided to follow my hunch and question her about the energy I felt in the room. I asked her if she ever imagined dancing with fairies? That strange pixie look came back as she looked at me with some surprise and admitted this was true! Following this metaphor, I said: 'I bet the fairies are falling about laughing because you have a "rock" stuck in your head! What if it was just a little fairy spell – maybe you could undo it if you were willing to love yourself. You'd probably find that the "rock" could turn back into a fairy!' Well, then she imagined looking inside the 'rock' and saw her little six-year-old self. And this little girl felt really guilty because she believed her closeness with her dad had interfered with her parents' relationship. So to make up for this, she had decided to be the BEST, and her whole focus became fierce perfectionism. In the process, she forgot how much she just loved to dance! It was all just a mistake.

As we talked about being in each moment and allowing 'the dance to dance you', instead of trying so hard to be the best, her internal conflict began to ease. She got to the place where she could just allow herself to be her unique self, able to allow the dance to come through her. She said when she danced she felt as light as the fairies she saw dancing around her. The 'rock' had diminished by then, so we invited it to become the centre of gravity in her belly that every dancer needs. This allowed her to come more fully back into her body and her headache began to ease a bit.

However, the remaining pain was still signalling something was not quite right. We talked about her frustration about not being able to realise her dreams. She had always been so good at planning her life, first to be a gymnast and then a dancer. Her control and will-power were evidence of how much she wanted it 'her way'. She admitted this was true. She had been positively obsessed with becoming a dancer for all these years. It was only recently that she had started considering that her life could be about anything else. I asked her: 'What if your soul purpose was much bigger than being a dancer? And what if the pain was just a signal that you are still trying to be too much in control?' Through her religious beliefs, she felt a strong connection to the Virgin Mary. So she chose to let go of the control and create a spiritual energy channel to Mary. Every time she felt any pain, she just sent the black pain up to Mary who transformed it into gold. She was astonished to feel her headache vanish completely for the first time she could remember.

How do you know if you are using too much control and will-power? Get suspicious when things are not going well, or not according to your plan. If you are feeling very frustrated that things have not gone your way, have a look at what your expectations have been. Rather like the old joke: 'How do you make God laugh?' Answer: 'Tell him your plans!' Instead of delineating exact details of what you want, dream your dream of the life script you would love to live. Let go of exactly how it will turn out.

> *For one who has conquered the mind, the mind is the best of friends. But for one who has failed to do so, his very mind will be his greatest enemy.*
>
> Bhagavad Gita

Designing Your Dream Script

Sometimes people have become so discouraged and disheartened they can't even begin to imagine what a positive life script could be for them. Maybe they've tried goal setting exercises before and it never made any difference. Maybe they are just so surrounded by things they perceive to be unchangeable that they cannot think beyond that, or imagine it could ever be any different. Sometimes just thinking about what they want makes them feel more depressed or even angry because of the difficult circumstances they are in. They have learned to accept the way things are, in order to cope, and they feel powerless to change anything. They don't believe anything they do will make a difference. If that is the case for you, read Chapters 4, 5 and 6 first to get a better understanding about what is happening now, before attempting to create your Dream Script.

Alternatively, sometimes the thought of too much change is daunting. Some people don't like change. They only feel safe and secure if things stay more or less the same. If that describes you, then you can still benefit if you start with smaller goals that you would like to achieve. You might find that adding together several smaller goals in different aspects of your life will allow you to change more gradually and carefully. Think of some specific outcomes that would improve your life, and bring you more happiness. As you succeed in making small changes, you may build enough courage to repeat the whole process and go for something bigger.

Don't limit yourself by thinking only of what other people have done. You might come up with something no one has ever thought of before! If you can, make sure what you put in your script is feasible as well as desirable. Is it possible for you to live this script? Do you have what it takes – in principle? Are you theoretically capable of maintaining all the aspects of living this script in real life? If you lived this script, would it hurt anyone or anything? Would the results of you achieving all your goals be ecologically friendly?

Do your best to avoid glib answers like winning the lottery or anything else that would be totally up to chance and nothing you could prepare for. Many people think that simply by having vast sums of money all their troubles will be over and they will be able to buy everything they ever wanted, give up their jobs, travel, and live a life of ease and pleasure. However, many people who win the lottery don't experience happiness. It isn't that easy. By all means include manifesting all the abundance you would like to have, but you will get more out of the exercises in this book if there are specific things you can do to create that abundance. Ask yourself: what would being rich allow you to do? Who will you be and what will you be doing then? Who will your friends be and how will you regard each other? What will be the effect on your family? How will you spend your time and energy?

Exercise: Creating your Dream Script ....
What would you like to have in your Dream Script?
1. Close your eyes and imagine or daydream your most positive scenario.
2. Step into it, in your mind's eye, and fully experience what it would be like.
3. What will you be seeing, hearing, feeling, doing, smelling,

tasting? What will you be saying to yourself? Where will you be?

4. Notice how you are feeling in this positive movie, and what you believe about yourself, about life. Who will you be?
5. Take a few moments to write down a short description of your Dream Script, or make a list of the main features.

N.B. It is very important to avoid making it specifically about a particular person, place or job, unless these are already part of your life. If you chose to imagine getting married to a specific person you are not yet in relationship with, for instance, that doesn't allow the universe the possibility of sending you someone who could be an even more perfect partner. Instead make it about the type of person, the qualities of a location, or the nature of some line of work, rather than something too specific.

Example: One client imagined creating a whole new life with a different career that involved travelling the world, doing archaeological work that was really exciting and rewarding, having an abundant income, a happy relationship, being 10 pounds lighter, much fitter, enjoying lots of fun holidays with friends, and learning how to scuba dive.

Deciding what you want, what will really make your heart sing, is the most important exercise in this book. What will make you want to jump out of bed in the morning because you just can't wait to do it? What will you find so fascinating that any time, effort or sweat you put into it feels like fun? What will attract you like a beacon, no matter how tough the journey to get there might be? What will make everything about your life feel worthwhile? What will make you feel excited enough to finish all the processes in this book so that your dream script can be a reality!

Chapter Summary:
Principles:
Begin with a positive outcome in mind.
The meaning of the communication is the response that you get.
Think big and stay flexible about your ideas for happiness.

Checklist:
1. Think big: dare to dream about what you really want.
   a. If you could be sure of success, what would you choose?
   b. If you knew you couldn't fail, what would you dare to do?
   c. If you were sure you could be happy, what would you change?
2. List all the activities and interests you love best, and include them in your Dream Script.
3. Score your current level of happiness: think of a number between 1–10
   a. How happy are you?
   b. How much effort are you making right now to create more happiness?
   c. If you can be objective, how successful have you been, so far?
4. Imagine and write down a Dream Script for your life.

2

A Recipe for Success

A man is about as happy as he makes up his mind to be.

ABRAHAM LINCOLN

Have you already noticed that your Dream Script has a certain flavour? Just like cooking up a new recipe, each ingredient you put in will make it that much more satisfying. Each person makes different choices, and their scripts have distinct qualities that make each one unique and special. Even though there may be time-honoured recipes that many people want to follow in their lives, no two scripts will be exactly the same. What is important is that you honestly get in touch with what you want, what is true for you rather than just following someone else's ideas, or some generalised notions of what constitutes a happy life. This may require heightening your senses.

When I first attended trainings in NLP (Neuro Linguistic Programming), what impressed me greatly about the best teachers, was their sensitivity when listening and communicating with each and every person. I had never seen people treat other people with so much respect and kindness. They seemed to have genuine curiosity about what the other person was thinking and feeling, instead of analysing or judging them. These teachers took great care to respond in a way that assisted people to find their own answers. They didn't pontificate or insist that other people adopt their ideas. They often used humour to help people see different perspectives and even laugh at their problems, yet they kept their feet firmly on the ground. Their ability to see more, hear more and understand more of what was going on, helped them coach people to discover their own solutions.

This attitude of sensitivity, and objective curiosity is an important element of compassionately coaching yourself as well as getting along with others. It's easy. All you have to do is resist the tendency to pre-judge a situation or a person. Instead, hold an open mind about how that person might be thinking and feeling. Remember that whatever they are doing makes perfect sense in their world. If you think about things you have said or done in the past, your actions usually made sense to you at the time. Even if you were making a mistake, there was usually a reason for that. Other people have reasons for being the way they are too.

It is important to realise that whatever you are thinking, doing and feeling right now in this moment is the best you are capable of. Even if you are making a mistake or feeling miserable, for whatever reasons, this is the best you can do at this moment in time. The total amount of knowledge that you have absorbed, your understanding, your education, your experience, your wounds, and your genetic make up, all add up to where you are right now. If it is less than perfect, all it means is that you still have more to learn. You can't do better than your best, but there is always room for improvement. Be patient and compassionate about your process of learning and growing.

Every Person has their own Map of the World

It helps to respect that there are different ways of thinking and viewing the world and to remember that everyone makes mistakes. Because you tend to hang out with people who think like you, sometimes it is easy to assume the way you see the world is the way everyone sees the world. You might be surprised to discover that other people have completely different ideas, beliefs and feelings to you, and that they have good reasons for being like that. If you can resist judging what is different, it can be interesting to learn about other people's strategies of thinking. Their solutions to problems might be better than yours!

It is also good to notice that a line of thinking may start with the best intentions and then go off track. What works in one situation, creates difficulties in another. Maybe you used to behave in a certain way and it got the results you wanted. But when you do that in a different context, it gets you into trouble, or it just doesn't produce the right results. Like a good detective, when you notice that the evidence shows there's a problem, trace it back to how your thinking may have contributed to that. Making a small adjustment to your ideas or behaviour can work magic.

Does your Dream Script include all major areas of your life? Make sure that there are scenes covering work, career, relationships, family, health, fitness, leisure, adventure, learning, development, creativity, contribution and even spiritual growth. This will ensure that you have been honest with yourself about all your most secret desires. Be thorough and imagine the best scenarios throughout your life. By getting in touch with your dreams, you will be able to discover your hidden goals and needs. At this point, think big! Later on you can become more specific about your Script as you think about each outcome more carefully.

What Flavour Is Your Story?

Have you ever noticed what makes a good story or a great movie? Aren't there usually difficulties in the present that eventually get resolved into an interesting outcome? Often there is a hero or heroine who struggles against the odds to achieve the impossible and then succeeds in the end. Are there ways you need to transcend whatever or wherever you are now, to achieve some future happiness? What is your particular style, or what kind of journey could provide the best path? Getting a sense of the flavour might help you know yourself better. This will make it easier to design successful strategies to manifest your Dream Script later on. What kind of positive outcome do you want? If you love adventure, better be sure that the journey you want to travel is packed with adventure! If you want a love story, you'd better be prepared to open your heart and really give your love.

Just imagine for the fun of it: what is the flavour of your Dream Script story? What kind of leading characters would you like to be with, and where is the action taking place? Does your Dream Script contain elements of:

- Adventure and exploration?
- Action-packed excitement?
- Love and transformation?

- Winning over the odds?
- Success story?
- Healing path?
- Hero epic?
- Detective novel?
- Epic travel journey?

How would you sum up the general flavour of your script? Quite often the type of books and magazines you read, movies you like to watch, or TV shows that grab your interest will also reflect the kind of Dream Script you've always wanted to live. Notice if you have a tendency to be attracted to a certain flavour of entertainment. The crucial elements of the story or the essence of the journey involved can help to clarify your direction and enhance your motivation to make it happen.

You must do the thing you think you cannot do.
Eleanor Roosevelt

A Big Dream

Anne chose to create a spiritual healing journey Script. On her sixtieth birthday, she decided life begins at sixty! Even though she had never had a formal career, her life so far had been rich and full. As the mother of three daughters with several grandchildren, and long divorced from her husband, now she felt it was time for something new. She dreamed of creating a centre in France where she could give back to the world what it had given to her. Her life story, so far, was already an inspiring journey of transformation. In order to manifest her new Dream Script, she would need a property big enough to receive groups as well as serve her family's needs. She wanted it to be a place where people would come for personal development workshops and where she could teach yoga, and write books. She was writing a book about her life experiences, and wanted an agent for her book. She was also looking for a publisher for another book about her grandfather. And she wanted a partner for perfect love. She would need to sell her house in London at a much higher price than the current market value to make all this possible. Playfully, I said that when her house in France was ready, I would be her first client!

Clearly, she was thinking big! Despite having been brought up to be a traditional wife and mother and never do 'important' things or have a career, she now had much bigger goals. Her whole education had been far away from any sort of accomplishment. So one of the major beliefs she had to change was that she couldn't do it. Instead she could recognise her purpose in life and then live it. Gradually, during the *Compassionate Coaching* process, she realised that she had all the skills she needed – they had always been there, waiting to be recognised. A smaller hurdle was that she wasn't yet a certified yoga teacher, but that was only a matter of finishing her training. Perhaps more importantly she needed much better communication skills – the way she was used to speaking didn't achieve the results she wanted. She had no idea how to get into rapport with people or how to understand another person's point of view. This was not helping her to achieve her plans. Training in *Compassionate Coaching* taught her many new skills and improved the way she both listened and expressed herself. She also found that she started thinking quite differently about people and became much less judgemental.

She was very clear and certain about what she wanted. What she needed to focus on was working through the beliefs and doubts that held her back. She also had to deal with the negative reactions of her whole family. They were not supportive of her plans because they worried that their inheritance would go down the drain. She also needed to learn to talk to herself without dragging herself down. In the past she used to become emotionally involved and anxious. Now she was able to let go, have faith, and allow Grace to help make things happen.

Just a few months later she found an ideal property in France, although it needed complete renovation. After selling her house for a very good price, she was able to put all her plans into action. She found the perfect builder who understood exactly what she wanted. He worked together with her over eighteen months to build the house of her dreams. Phase 1 took six months, with two of the buildings made habitable for her family at Christmas.

A year later, she hosted her first group workshop – yes, it was one of my training seminars! Not long after that, she became a certified yoga teacher and started teaching her own classes. She found the agent and publisher for her books, and her Manoir became a centre for all kinds of different personal development workshops and exhibitions. Because of the changes in world finances, her family now appreciated that her investment in building this incredible property was a very shrewd move benefiting everyone. She achieved her dreams!

The Trap of Being Impatient

Many people get very impatient and want to achieve their results immediately. No sooner have they thought of an idea, than they want to jump into action without doing enough assessment and preparation. They start putting all their energy into activities that might be a waste of time. They may not have even checked to be sure that their outcome is what they truly want. Jumping into action too soon can actually lead you up blind alleys. This book is carefully designed to make sure you don't miss any important steps or considerations. If you follow the directions and complete the exercises, your Dream Script should be thoroughly prepared, and have the best possible chance to easily become a reality.

Sometimes people haven't checked out whether they really want what they think they want. Or worse, they are already anticipating how it won't work, so then they talk themselves out of it and give up without even trying. They may have one of those cynical internal voices that talks to them all day long about how things won't work out. This may be just an old habit, going back to childhood when someone told them they were no good at doing something. If you have one of those voices that gets in the way of thinking positively here are several different ways to deal with it. Imagine you have an internal remote control:

- Turn the volume down.
- Change the channel to one you enjoy listening to.
- Introduce an imaginary interruptive noise, like a gong to chime in whenever this voice starts bothering you.

- Change the quality of the voice: allow it to say whatever it wants, but make it sound like a sexy movie star, or a cartoon character.
- Move the location of the voice to your left big toe or your elbow or some other distant place. Let it speak from there.

Doesn't it sound different? With practice, using your remote control can help clear your head so that you can think more objectively.

It may be that people have told you since you were very young that you had certain talents or capabilities, and therefore you should do 'X'. You may have accepted that without questioning the decision. You may have made all your education and career decisions based on what other people said, and never stopped to properly evaluate what you wanted to do. Or maybe after you achieved a certain level of success, you just felt ready to move on to something new. It might be time to reconsider where you are now, and what it is you really want now. Your wants and needs change with time. Are the outcomes in your Dream Script:

- Up-to-date?
- Your own desires rather than other people's wishes?
- Designed to take you where you want to go in the future?

Another way impatience manifests itself is through being overly solution oriented. Have you ever noticed how much energy you spend trying to fix things? Our whole culture seems to be obsessed with being clever, quick witted, and sounding intelligent. You are supposed to get smart and figure things out, identify the problem and implement the solution. There's a belief that success depends on applying the right analytical ability in all situations. If you are not getting the goals you want, then there must be some missing knowledge, something you need to learn or some action to take right now.

This kind of thinking may have motivated you to read this book! Reading self-help books, going on workshops, seeing therapists, getting coaching etc. are all ways of trying to find the missing answers and solutions. Isn't it fortunate that there are now many good sources where you can discover answers that will help you learn and gain greater wisdom. The intention of this book is to help you channel your acquired wisdom into an easy process that actually works. Then all your wisdom can be put to good use.

Unfortunately some people get lost and confused when they start looking for the answers. They end up stuck in their heads, often using the very tools they've learned to beat themselves up even more. They become adept at describing their problem from every angle. Despite analysing all the aspects of it, the problem doesn't shift and the desired results do not happen. Then they feel even more of a failure than before they started. It is important to keep your sense of humour and take everything lightly. If things haven't changed yet, there's probably a very good reason. 'God's delays are not God's denials' is a phrase that helps many people put this in perspective. You may not know yet why things haven't changed, but in the meantime, make this delay an opportunity for learning even more.

If you listen to the chatter that goes on in your mind during the day, notice if you are spending too much energy judging, thinking, reasoning, analysing or just going over and over and over a situation that you haven't been able to resolve. If you haven't managed to come up with the solution, then it is more than likely that this type of thinking will never come up with the solution. Do something completely different! Change the channel of your mind by changing your behaviour. Do something active, exercise, dance, get involved with some kind of creative activity. Using your body can help change your perspective. Just going for a walk and appreciating nature, works wonders sometimes. By accessing different parts of your mind, new solutions are more likely to appear spontaneously.

Healing Obsession

The type of thinking that keeps you stuck in a problem is not the type of thinking that can get you out of it. Sometimes the problem begins with being too attached to the result you want, making it too important. A classic example was a young divorcee who really wanted to have a new relationship, but it just wasn't happening. She was very clear about what she wanted. She had listed all the qualities of her ideal partner. She was really good at getting 'out there' and meeting potential partners, but often found they were not as interested as she was. After being rejected and hurt quite a number of times, her desire to find true love was becoming eclipsed by her fear of losing any love she might find. She began feeling very inadequate.

She started demonstrating 'learned helplessness' just like the rats in psychology experiments, where the scientists electrified different squares on the floor of the cage. When the rats touched various squares they received a shock. Gradually the rats just stayed still to avoid the shocks as they had learned that nothing they could do would make a difference. A part of her started to believe that she wasn't supposed to have a relationship. No matter what she did, it never seemed to make a difference. In fact, she said that her life worked so well now, that she couldn't imagine how any man could add to it! This part of her didn't want to lose any of her freedom or add the extra hassle of having to deal with someone else's issues. But even as she said this, the other part of her that was so attached to having a relationship retorted that she would NOT give up or give in! And so her internal battle continued.

What happens when you want a goal or outcome too much? It can become an obsession, something you need so much that it is like an addiction. Whenever you want something so much, ironically you keep that very thing away. When you want something, you are focusing on what you lack. By focusing on what you lack, what you don't allow yourself to have, you perpetually maintain the situation via the pictures you make in your mind. Putting your energy into the wanting effectively robs you of your ability to manifest a good result. Whenever you say you want something, it sounds like you are stating a goal, but in fact, you are stating what you have not yet allowed yourself to have.

The paradox is that if you can let go of the wanting and the neediness, then you can easily have anything. A curious dynamic of life is that you can only have what you don't need. Equally, what you resist, persists. So if all your energy is being used to get your needs met, and to avoid whatever you fear, that creates an effective strategy for disappointment. Either your attachment, expectations and demands push away the very thing you want, or your avoidance of whatever you fear attracts the very thing you don't want. When it no longer matters whether you have it or not, then you can just manifest what is true for you. But when you get caught in wanting something too much, it can feel close to impossible to let go. What's the way out of this?

What helps is to shift your perspective and think logically from a completely different angle. The easy way to do this is to step out of the dynamic for minute. Remember that you are much more than this internal conflict. It may have been consuming all your energy and your mind might have been obsessing about it day and night. Shift your awareness to your heart instead. Breathe into your heart until you calm down. Let your heart guide you. Listen to what your heart has to say and be willing to follow that advice.

Notice that when you want something too much, it actually emphasises the message that you lack that very thing. 'Well, obviously,' you might say! The evidence of not having it is clear. But the problem is that all your energy is supporting the lack, which fuels the neediness. When you are needy it is difficult, if not impossible, to receive. In fact, even if success comes your way, you're more likely to sabotage it. You will make demands, look for faults, or even push it away, whether you perceive it to be good enough or not good enough.

Imagine there is a camcorder filming every moment of your entire life, every movement you make and even the narrative of your internal thoughts and experiences. What positive qualities would this camera pick up about who you are, how you are feeling and what your life story is all about? Maybe you have been too embroiled in one scene or with one potential outcome of this story. Maybe the whole tale is much richer and more mysterious than you could ever imagine. What if there were other potential outcomes that could be even better than the one you have been chasing?

Putting her life back into a more balanced perspective, and remembering who she was, allowed this young divorcee to re-access her heart and feel more present. She stopped over-focusing on her desired outcome. As she accepted herself more, she relaxed and chose to consider her outcome as more of a direction. This allowed her to be more flexible and curious about letting things unfold. She even felt more trusting again. She felt open and easy about a new relationship.

In case you are wondering how to know if you are obsessing about a particular outcome or result that you want, there's an easy way to tell. Score yourself out of ten: 'How much are you still focused on wanting things to be different?' If you are not feeling relaxed about whether or not it ever happens, you may still be too attached. You are unattached if:

- It is OK whether or not you succeed in having this outcome.
- You can let go and frame a new goal easily.
- You can learn from the experience and move on.

If you are obsessing about a particular outcome, just do your best to let go. There are useful exercises later on to help free up attachment.

If you do not need anything from another person, you cannot be pushed away.

Chuck Spezzano

Your Dream Script Reveals Your Goals

Now that you have a full picture of what your Dream Script looks like, and you know what flavour it is, it is time to get quite specific. When you assess each aspect of your Script, you might notice that your story incorporates many goals that you might not have ordinarily thought of. This is the beauty of thinking big and creating a Dream Script. You can get in touch more accurately with unconscious goals, needs and motivations. It is a good idea now to be precise about what you want. Then you can more accurately assess what will help you to achieve it, and what holds you back. As you consider your Dream Script, extract all the goals that will be achieved when you are living it in real life. Some goals might be obvious, some more implicit. Find out what you want to have happen specifically:

Exercise: What are your specific goals? ....

Consider the following categories one by one:

Work and career: how would you like to develop your work?
Relationships: how would you like to improve your intimate relationships?
Family: what might need to be healed, appreciated or changed?
Health and fitness: could your diet or exercise routines be better?
Leisure: how well balanced are your work and home life?
Adventure: are you challenged enough or do you need more excitement?
Learning and development: in what ways would you like to grow and learn?
Creativity: are you yearning to develop some creative talent?
Contribution: what would you like to give?
Spiritual growth: what deeper issues might you need to resolve?

1. As you imagine living your Dream Script, think about each of these categories, and write down some specific goals your script reveals for each area, stating them in present tense, for example:
   I am. . . . . .
   I have. . . . .
   I'm doing. . . . . .
   I'm feeling. . . . . .
   I'm looking. . . . . .
   I'm seeing, hearing, smelling, tasting. . . . .
   I'm moving to. . . . . .
   I'm giving. . . . .
   I'm receiving. . . . .
2. Notice which goals are most important to you. Perhaps put stars next to the most important ones, or re-list them in order of importance.
3. Check that these goals are all possible and potentially achievable.
4. If any of them are impossible for you, adjust the goals or your script as necessary to write your story with goals that are potentially possible.

5. How much would you like these goals to happen? Notice how much energy you have already invested in each one. You might even like to score each one out of ten to compare how motivated you feel right now.

....

Hidden Needs

When your goals are not happening naturally, it may be that you want them too much and can't let go. Whenever you get stuck on wanting something too much, your neediness could repel that very thing. But what is it that keeps us so stuck? Often there are hidden deeper needs underneath the wanting too much that fuels the attachment. There must be a belief that somehow, whatever it is you want so badly will satisfy one of these deeper hidden needs. Although it is normal to have these needs, sometimes they can prevent you from doing what you want, or propel you in directions you'd rather not go, or just silently keep you stuck repeating the same old problems again and again.

A Hidden Need for Acceptance, Control and Safety

A successful banker had finally found the woman of his dreams – he thought. The relationship seemed to be flourishing over several months and he began to start thinking very seriously about commitment. Suddenly his girlfriend decided to end it, for no apparent reason. Obviously she had been thinking along very different lines. The banker was shocked. He kept obsessing about how right they were for each other, how good it could be and what a mistake it was to end it. He couldn't let go. In fact, he felt quite angry and frustrated at not getting what he wanted. Even worse, this was not the first time this had happened in his life.

He felt that somehow he often left women feeling frustrated. He wanted to be there, but he always held something back from them. He was afraid of committing to someone and later regretting it. Now after being burnt so many times, he was beginning to believe that it wasn't safe to share his heart at all. What could be the cause of this he wondered? At school, he had been teased by the other students for not being good enough. But he could never work out how or why. More recently he noticed a pattern of not feeling accepted by various groups. So underneath his desire for a committed relationship, could there be a deeper belief system about needing to be accepted and loved? In fact, this hit a nerve! As he got in touch with his deeper hidden lack of love and acceptance, he felt quite angry.

The frustration he felt about never having received a sense of love and acceptance had been with him all his life. He remembered being like this in his childhood. He even imagined being born feeling angry about it! In his birth story he saw himself feeling so helpless, confused and frustrated, just wanting the process of his birth to be over. He wanted to be in control, he couldn't feel the love from his mother, didn't feel he was accepted, and didn't trust anything that was happening. He felt this set the scene for many beliefs and decisions that were later amplified throughout his upbringing.

During his session, he imagined being able to access his heart and from this wise and compassionate perspective, he delivered some better ideas to the little baby as he was being born. He gave him reassurance that: 'Things would be all right in the end. It's OK to trust. Trust has no pre-conditions. He can rely on love, even when he can't see or feel it. It is better to go with the flow.' As he felt the truth of each idea for himself, he imagined the baby relaxing and letting go. The deep layer of belief about needing acceptance, control and safety was released, allowing him to access his inner truth about his natural abundance of love and acceptance.

Whenever you forget what is true for you, you lose contact with your wise inner heart centre. Deep inside is a place where each person is as complete and whole as a newborn baby. There is no lack, no guilt, no anger and no fear. You can remember to return there just as easily as you forget its existence. All it requires is a choice and a willingness to let go of what you judge to be fearful and lacking. This man did such a good job of letting go, that only a few months later, he found himself in a new

relationship with a woman who was even more wonderful than
the one who had rejected him.

> *It is still up to you to choose*
> *To join with truth or with illusion*
> *But remember that to choose one*
> *Is to let the other go.*

A Course in Miracles

The goals throughout your Dream Script can be extremely
useful in revealing hidden needs. Knowing what these needs
are and how these needs motivate you towards trying to achieve
certain outcomes, can set you free. As long as you are alive,
you will have needs. Your need for air, water, warmth, light and
nourishment are indisputable. Babies will not survive without
love and touch. To be healthy, you also need exercise and rest.
Aside from these basic needs, however, most of your other needs
will probably fall into one of three main categories: Love, Control
and Survival. Listening to thousands of clients has revealed that
these three types of needs are extremely common. The important point to remember, however, is that there is nothing
innately bad about having any of these needs. It's just useful
information that can help you to identify old patterns that might
still be holding you back.

Exercise: What are your hidden needs? ....
Look over each of your goals and determine which of these
three basic needs it satisfies: Love, Control or Survival.

Love: is your goal about getting acceptance, approval, respect,
acknowledgement, admiration, affirmation, esteem, appreciation, recognition, reassurance, belonging, closeness, companionship, consideration, empathy, fame, affection, intimacy,
feeling included, loved, cared for, important, cherished etc.,
possibly even enlightenment or transcendence.

Control: is your goal about having authority, position, power,
making decisions, making things happen, getting others to

co-operate or support you, having things your way, perfectionism, pushing, manipulating, proving your abilities or prowess,
insisting on rules or proper behaviour, order, beauty, symmetry,
being right, demanding, needing clarity, understanding, knowledge, structure, certainty, or completion.

Survival: is your goal about safety, security, creating space,
maintaining your boundaries, defence, protecting your vulnera-
bility, self esteem, feelings, space, freedom, self expression, or
your body. Creating abundance in order to meet all your
needs, saving, investing, healing, or overcoming obstacles and
risks, establishing your independence, autonomy or solidarity.

When you have reviewed each goal and determined what hidden
needs are being served, which category of needs predominates?
At this point, just notice what kind of needs you are fulfilling in
your script – this might reveal important patterns of behaviour
during the exercises later on in the book. There may be more
than one need in each goal. Sometimes they combine. Just note
any patterns that might emerge. You may begin to notice that
your current life, too, reflects attempts to get these needs met.

*Example: One client had a rich life script that contained many
different goals. Her three most important ones were: to change
her career to become a Life Coach, to meet and marry the man
of her dreams, and to buy a house in the country. As she
thought about 'I am now working as a Life Coach', she realised
this goal was about her having more control over her work, her
time and her fulfilment. 'I am now married to the man of my
dreams' was about getting love, affection, companionship and
intimacy. 'I now live in a beautiful house in the country' was
about security, space and abundance. As she became more
aware of her hidden needs, she was able to focus more easily
on how to begin fulfilling them right now, and also to appreciate
all the ways she was already enjoying some of those qualities.*

These hidden needs usually sound like good qualities. Most of
them are common, normal needs that most people have or do

their best to get fulfilled. As balanced principles of behaviour, when there is no attachment present, these three needs present no problem at all. But when they trigger neediness and obsessive behaviour, or unconscious energies of compulsion or repulsion, then they are no longer good qualities to have fuelling your Script. In later chapters, you will learn how to use these needs to direct you to a healing solution. Then it will be possible to have the need as a balanced quality without any attachment.

If you notice that many of your goals are attempts to get one particular need met, that could be a clue. Perhaps a part of you feels that you've never had that need met. When you lacked something in the past, it is quite natural to dream about a future script where you finally have all the ingredients for happiness.

You might be surprised to discover that your goals have something to do with healing old wounds from the past and putting things to rights. Sometimes if there has been a problem in your past history, you might have felt propelled in the opposite direction in an attempt to avoid such a thing ever happening again. Or you might find that, without realising it, you are following the mistaken guidance of some role model in your past and continuing to make the same mistakes again. It can be humbling to realise how much of your time and energy is already engaged in trying to meet these unmet needs from the past. Unfortunately, these hidden needs can be quite compelling. Once again, it is useful to maintain your sense of humour. Smile indulgently at yourself whenever you find you've engaged in compulsive behaviour in order to get one of these needs fulfilled. 'Oh, isn't that cute, I'm doing it again!' In later chapters, you will learn how to make a better choice.

Once you have identified your goals, and the hidden needs behind them, you may want to adjust your Dream Script. You can do that at any time, but it is important to re-do the steps that have been covered so far with any new Script that you might create. When you have your Dream Script ready, the next step will be to discover your purpose: knowing who you are and what you want to contribute by being here in this life. Your purpose is the single, most powerful, motivating factor in propelling you into making the right decisions. When you have your purpose guiding everything you do, choosing the right moves is easy. No matter what is happening, your purpose will act as a steadying influence, supporting you through any challenges you might meet along your path. It will be your measuring stick for evaluating choices, and making changes. In the next chapter, you can easily discover your purpose through identifying your gifts.

Chapter Summary:
Principles:
Every person has their own map of the world.
The person with the most flexibility of behaviour has the highest probability of achieving the results they desire.
Let go of attachments.

Checklist
1. Does your script include all major areas of your life?
   - Work
   - Career
   - Relationships
   - Family
   - Health
   - Fitness
   - Leisure
   - Adventure
   - Learning
   - Development
   - Creativity
   - Contribution
   - Spiritual growth
2. What flavour is your script?
   - Adventure and exploration
   - Action-packed excitement
   - Love and transformation
   - Winning over the odds
   - Success story
   - Healing path
   - Hero epic
   - Detective novel
   - Epic travel journey

3. What are all your positive goals that it reveals?
   List each of your goals stated in the positive.
4. Are the outcomes in your Dream Script:
   • Up-to-date?
   • Your own desires rather than other people's wishes?
   • Designed to take you where you want to go in the future?
5. Dealing with internal dialogue:
   • Turn the volume down
   • Change the quality of the voice: allow it to say whatever it wants, but make it sound like a sexy movie star, or a cartoon character.
   • Move the location of the voice to your left big toe. Let it speak from there
6. Are you attached to your outcome?
   • Is it OK whether or not you succeed in having this outcome?
   • Can you let go and frame a new goal easily?
   • Have you learned from experience and moved on?
7. What are the underlying needs those goals are trying to fulfil?
   • Love and Appreciation
   • Being in Control
   • Safety and Security

3

What is Your Gift?

What lies behind us and lies before us are small matters compared to what lies within us. And when we bring what is within us out into the world, miracles happen.

HENRY DAVID THOREAU

When you think about the best moments in your life so far, are they the moments when you are excelling or giving your best? Do you think about standing in wonder appreciating beauty in some way? Are they times when you are surrounded by people you love, basking in the good feelings, laughter and fun? Or perhaps a precious instant of feeling awe while experiencing the perfection of someone you love, even yourself, or the world? Your best moments may be unique and different from anyone else's, and these are usually times when you are sharing your most special gifts.

When you think about being talented or gifted, most people think of musicians, singers, actors, artists, dancers or icons of sport. When someone demonstrates an extraordinary talent in a particular field, it is easy to perceive that as a gift. But many other gifts go unrecognised because they are more personal, more of the moment. For instance, you can have great talent for being considerate, determined, or relaxed. Your gift might be something that just makes you someone everyone likes to be around. Your gift might be lighting up the room with your energy when you walk in, and brightening people's day. Your talent might inspire and empower others. As you think about living your Dream Script, what gifts or talents will you be demonstrating by who you are? What energy will you be giving? What passion will you be sharing?

Giving Yourself

Sometimes your particular gift might be how you appreciate the wonders of the world. It might be your fascination with nature, history, archaeology, or some other special field of study. Are there special interests you'd like to pursue in your Dream Script? What could make you feel passionately alive, energised, enthusiastic and happy? What gifted qualities will you have when you become the person of your Dream Script?

Your talents might not be singing, playing a musical instrument or creating some work of art. Your special gifts may be more about how you share yourself, your energy, or how you contribute in your own unique way. Here is a sample list of particular talents to get you thinking more broadly:

Adventurousness
Affirming what is good
Appreciation
Beauty
Bringing harmony
Buoyancy
Caring for others
Celebration and excitement
Closeness and intimacy
Compassion and love
Co-operation, collaboration
Confidence
Consideration
Courage
Curiosity
Determination
Diligence
Directness or clarity of mind
Enthusiasm
Establishing order
Excelling as an example
Finding meaning
Finishing things, completion
Freshness and light heartedness
Generosity

Getting things started
Giving
Good communication
Gratitude
Having a balanced view
Helping people belong
Helping people grow
Honesty and truth
Humility
Humour, fun and play
Imagination
Innocence
Intuition
Inspiring others
Joy
Kindness
Luck
Moving forward
Nurturing
Openness
Patience
Peace
Precision
Quick wit
Relaxation
Showing what is possible
Standing up for freedom
Teamwork
Tenderness
Understanding
Variety
Vision
Willingness

Example: The woman who wanted to be a Life Coach realised she had many gifts to give: appreciation of other people's gifts, compassion, confidence, consideration, determination, directness, enthusiasm, good communication, humour, intuition, patience, and understanding.

The list is as endless as there are human beings on the planet. Everyone has unique gifts to give. Perhaps your gifts are part of your purpose for being here. The hologram of the world would not be complete or perfect without you and your gifts. How well you deliver and share your gifts, though, is your choice.

While reviewing your script, can you identify specifically what natural talents, interests, abilities, and gifts you really want to be giving? Put a special tick mark next to all the qualities that you already do give. What will you continue to give in even better ways when you live your Dream Script? Remember to appreciate how much you have to give, and how much you have already given just by being you.

Exercise: What are your gifts? ....

Identify all your natural talents, interests or gifts that you already give and will be giving in your ideal script. You could start with ticking the list above.

1. What gifts do you give to your most intimate partner and family?
2. What talents do you share through your work or hobbies?
3. What natural capabilities, or qualities make you great to work with?
4. What gifts do you give to your friends? What do you give yourself?
5. How do you bring enjoyment into the world?
6. What interests, or special projects, or causes do you invest your time in?
7. How do you inspire others or set an example?
8. What do you give just by being present?

....

You may be surprised to discover just how many gifts you already bring into the world. Why not start appreciating now, just how special you are in your own unique way? By starting with an attitude of gratitude for all your positive qualities, talents and gifts, you are more likely to create a magnetic force that draws more good qualities towards you. The better you feel about who and where you are now, the easier it will be to change and improve. Even if you are currently feeling low, at least you are brave enough to explore the depths! Sometimes, when you are in a black mood, it is hard to think positively about having any good qualities at all. At times like that, it can be helpful to have a friend or coach do a more objective assessment.

Sometimes having too many gifts and talents can feel like a burden. Do you feel obligated to do them all? You might already be giving so much in so many different ways that you fear you will become exhausted. Have you forgotten to give enough to yourself? Maybe you've left yourself out of the equation. Why not take a moment now and commit to nourish yourself. What can you do on a daily basis to keep yourself in balance? In your Dream Script be sure to include ways to give to yourself, so that you give from a place of inner abundance.

When you are multi-talented and want to choose a new career direction, how do you focus on one path? Which talents or gifts will you choose and which ones will be put aside? Could you create some kind of portfolio career? Are there enough hours in each day and enough energy to put into each one or will they all get short-changed? If you push to do too much, you could risk burnout and exhaustion.

To have clear goals and put all your effort into achieving your objectives is a proven recipe for success. However, sometimes focusing too much on the desired result can pull you off your centre. You can be too conscientious! Burnout feels like a physical phenomenon because both your mind and body get exhausted. On a deeper level, it's mistaken thinking that leads to driving yourself beyond what is physically endurable. It isn't just high-flying executives who suffer burnout. It can also happen at any age, as the following story illustrates.

How can I go forward when I don't know which way I'm facing?

John Lennon

Exhaustion and Burnout

A mother sent her teenage son to see me. Despite being extremely clever, charming and doing quite well at school, he felt terribly tired and exhausted most of the time. He also didn't seem to fit in very well with the other boys because he didn't like sports. So he spent most of his spare time playing with computers.

When I questioned him about his tiredness, he merely said it was due to having to study so hard for exams. All he really enjoyed doing was playing with his computer at home and not going out anywhere. It seemed an effort for him to even answer my questions. He told me that he had been sent to psychiatrists regularly since he was very young. His mother had told me that his birth had been very difficult and painful for her. Consequently, she had never bonded with this boy, and just couldn't love him as much as her other son and daughter.

As we talked, I noticed his eyes were fixed on a position down to his right. So I asked him what he was looking at. Surprisingly, he said 'A beach'. He was running a movie of an idealised beach, where people were playing and having a good time. He imagined running about with the waves and discovering all kinds of shells, fish, crabs and sea creatures. As he described it, he admitted feeling sad. There was such a contrast between his hard-working life and that beautiful beach. He felt that his whole existence was a struggle to prove that he was good enough and worthy of being loved.

He also wanted to be like his father who worked from home and had lots of free time to pursue his hobby of flying. His father often spent long hours helping his clients and was incredibly diligent and serious. I could tell by the way he talked about him, that he really admired his father. In fact, it was quite likely he was a chip off the old block. He probably had absorbed his father's beliefs and attitudes as well as inheriting his genetic disposition.

This hard-working script dictated that he would have to behave like his father in order to be successful. But secretly he longed to remain a carefree child who was free to play. Instead, he drove himself like a slave driver striving to do well in all his subjects to please everyone. He also worried about the career choices he had to make. How could he decide which subjects to major in at university? What would happen if he made the wrong choice? As he looked towards his future, it seemed like the rest of his life would be nothing but hard work. No wonder he felt so depressed, exhausted and burnt out.

Remembering the image of the beach, I asked him what the message of that fantasy could be? What fascinated him about being in that beautiful environment, exploring, discovering things, and having fun? Oddly enough, he looked down at his hands as he talked about how he loved to pick things up and hold them in his hands, and how that made him feel happy and connected with his world. I asked him how he could possibly bring some of that energy into his school work? Would it be possible to think about his studies as if they were an exploration of new worlds full of new ideas to pick up and hold, and how that could be fun? What if each subject was a different kind of beach, waiting to be discovered? This idea intrigued him.

We talked about how much more fun it would be if he listened to his heart, followed his heart, and then put his heart into everything that he did. What if he let his heart lead his head instead of using so much will power to override his feelings. Of course, when your heart is in what you are doing, it feels like play. I talked to him about being true to who he is. He protested that he didn't know who he was! But gradually he understood that he had the rest of his life to discover who he was, and that although he might make mistakes, everything he chose to experience would be an important part of his journey. He promised to take better care of the little child who wanted to play on the beach, by listening to what his heart really wanted, and taking time off to play. He began to understand that it was important to be kind to himself first.

Without love, the acquisition of knowledge only increases confusion and leads to self-destruction.

J. Krishnamurti

The Trap of Overwhelm

Your talents and gifts are some of the most powerful resources that will help you to manifest the script of your dreams. Think of a time you were experiencing joy, wonder, pleasure and delight whilst giving one of your gifts. Notice how effortless it felt! When you are giving what you love best, that energy creates ease, flow, and pleasure. Time seems to go with you instead of against you. You neither race the clock nor count the minutes going by. When you are giving your gifts, you are never stressed or bored. It feels natural. Whatever you do seems to come through you instead of something that you have to work at. It is almost a sense that you don't have to do anything at all except be present, with the intention of giving your best. Imagine being able to apply that kind of energy to creating the script of your dreams.

When you dream big plans, when you have massive ambition, when you want to be a huge success, you can feel excited and motivated. Your positive energy can also enthuse everyone around you. You'll find it easy to propel yourself into action, tap into phenomenal energy, and go for it! It can feel so good! You find it's easy to overcome obstacles, learn new skills, and deal with any problems . . . unless you hit overwhelm!

Some people hit overwhelm right after they think of a great idea. Their minds run old scripts that tell them they can't do it, it's impossible, they are not good enough and then they find they can't even get started. Some people forget their natural gifts and talents. They haven't remembered to tap into their creative flow or give their gifts. They forget how easy it becomes when you are just giving your best because you love doing what you are doing. Maybe that great idea wasn't really appropriate in their Dream Script. Perhaps it was something they thought would bring them happiness because other people do it, but maybe they forgot to check out that it was a true path in their own heart. It is always good to remember that it doesn't really matter what you do. What is important is that you love what you do. You could be sweeping the streets and be blissfully happy and fulfilled. What counts is the state you are in – the way you feel inside, and whether you are giving yourself in a true way.

Overwhelm differs from procrastination in that the job in question is something that is really desirable to do rather than something to avoid. People who procrastinate can suffer feelings of overwhelm when they let the jobs pile up so high that it requires superhuman effort to get anything done. But even though the tasks may be undesirable, when the time runs out and the deadlines threaten, they usually do the job.

People suffer from overwhelm when they have set themselves a huge objective, a goal that is so important and so big that it daunts them. What lurks behind overwhelm can be the fear of failure. Sometimes the expectations they put on themselves become a problem. How will they be able to deal with their own or other people's measure of success? Who will they have to compete with? What will they think of themselves if they don't make it?

Ironically, some people are more frightened of success than of failure. They imagine a fantastic Dream Script and doubt that they could handle being so successful. Do they really have the talents and skills to achieve their dreams or will they be exposed as frauds? Do they really deserve to be that well thought of, that abundant? Will they become someone they don't like? Will they get big headed? What if they can't maintain their course – what will happen if they reach success and then crash? How embarrassing that would be! Better to stay small and not even try.

A young, experienced film and TV editor wanted career advice because he was running an overwhelm script. No matter how motivated he felt towards his own private film project, he just couldn't finish it! He had spent years writing and filming it, but now it had sat for over five weeks waiting to be edited. It would never make the deadline for Cannes! He said with some sadness, 'When it's finally finished, after all the time and effort I've put into it, plus what other people have put into it, I'm afraid it won't be as good as I expect it to be. And other people may not think well of it either.' And so he froze into non-action. It was easier to keep his head under the duvet and dream. 'It all gets too confusing,' he said. 'Too many things to deal with, like a train stopping at forty stations. I can see it all OK, but when I go to do it, it's too big!'

Although he'd never been a failure in his life, and his family was very supportive, things never came easily for him. He was the oldest son, and his father had always said he should do whatever he really wanted to do . . . but make sure it is a success! He competed with his younger brother, who now seemed to be outshining him with great career success, a happy marriage and a new baby. The better his brother did, the higher his expectations for himself became and the more massive his ambition grew. He had to really excel just to be equal!

When we started to work with his 'Overwhelm Script', we suddenly hit resistance. He discovered a ten-year-old part of him that didn't want him to change, because it had a hidden need. It was keeping him 'safe'. He explained that, 'It keeps me from climbing trees that I might fall out of.' But this positive intention of safety had created a life of constant confusion, unhappiness and consequent panic attacks – which was worse than falling out of a tree! He decided to change his thinking about this. As an adult, he knew he could prepare himself adequately, take some risks and deal with the consequences. Once we were able to resolve his need for safety, we discovered that this 'Overwhelm Script' had been running in his family for at least three generations. Since it was a family habit, no wonder it had been hard for him to change it.

It seemed to start with his great grandfather: a successful young man who had a good job, but who was very unhappy. He worked so hard, he never got to see much of his family. Events forced him to stay stuck in this job, even though he wanted to do something completely different. He was unable to change and felt overwhelmed by the workload as much as the disappointment. He wasn't following his heart, but he feared that he would never succeed at doing what he really wanted to do. This pattern had been repeated with each generation, until now.

I asked the young film editor what positive beliefs might have helped his great grandfather? In no time at all, his heart was giving all kinds of advice: that there were so many options and choices, that no matter how hard it gets, something will make it right. That he should follow his instinct, be true to himself, ignore what other people think, even if it required a radical change to be who he came to be. And he also needed to change his definition of success from money and material possessions, to what he believes makes a person really happy, strong and enthusiastic.

These positive ideas were the perfect antidote for his own overwhelm, of course. In no time at all he was surprised to hear himself saying, 'Let me at it!' He couldn't wait to get back into action to edit his film. Since he had lots of ideas and contacts, all it required was to clarify his priorities and stay connected with his strength and enthusiasm.

Many persons have a wrong idea of what constitutes true happiness.
It is not attained through self-gratification
But through fidelity to a worthy purpose.

Helen Keller

Discovering Your Purpose

Your talents and gifts are closely related to your purpose. Your purpose may be simple, it may be grand, it may be highly spiritual or very practical. Just imagine that your soul or your spirit has a reason for being. What could be your purpose for being alive in this life? Have you ever considered how you hold a unique space in this corner of the universe? Just like every blade of grass and every grain of sand has its place, so do you. The universe would not be whole and complete without you. What is your special and unique function? What role do you play?

Knowing your purpose can be like having the most wonderful tour guide helping you to enjoy your journey. It can keep you on track, and steady you when the going gets rough. It can enrich your appreciation of every detail and every path that you explore. Following your purpose invites an incredible sense of grace to assist everything you do. Your purpose incorporates all your gifts, and permeates all your giving. It can supply that wonderful sense of meaning and fulfilment you've always wanted. If you don't already know what your purpose is, the following process can help you discover it, or put it into words. You may have more than one purpose, of course. There are many levels of purpose. There could be an immediate practical purpose behind what you do, but above that there may be a higher purpose you were not aware of. In the next exercise, you can discover your Highest Purpose, which quietly directs the delivery of all your gifts through everyday actions.

Exercise: Discover your purpose. ....

1. Take one of the most important goals that you have listed in your script and write it in the grey box marked Outcome. Ask yourself the question above the box, and place your answer in the 'Outcome 2' box. Ask the next question and place the answer in box 3. Keep repeating the same questioning until you can no longer go any higher. (Add more boxes if necessary)

2. Then repeat this procedure with some of your other goals. You will probably begin to see some similarities in your answers.

3. When you find similar or compatible answers, put them together into a sentence. This can reveal some of your gifts, and your Purpose.

Keep repeating questioning until you reach the highest outcome

⇧

If you got [Outcome 3] what would this allow you to do or be? [Outcome 4]

⇧

If you got [Outcome 2] what would this give you? [Outcome 3]

⇧

If you got this what would it do for you? [Outcome 2]

OUTCOME: What do you want?

4. Safety check: what would happen if you did live your Purpose and deliver your gifts? What else would have to change in your life? Would this be OK? How would this affect others? What would change for the whole planet if you delivered your gifts and lived your Purpose?
5. Take the Purpose statement you created, and consider your gifts. How will you be delivering your Purpose through the many various gifts that you have come to give? How are you already doing that?
6. You can make a personal Purpose statement and refine it until you are comfortable with how it sounds. It should be something you feel really good about, something that is very true about you. You may or may not wish to keep your purpose private and sacred. But the more you use it to remind yourself of your true path, the more powerful an influence it will begin to exert in your life.

Example: The woman who wanted to be a Life Coach chose to work on her goal of meeting and marrying the man of her dreams. She wrote this goal in the grey box. Then she asked herself what would this give her once she was happily married? The answer she put in the box above was: Fun, support, balance and growth. Then she asked herself what having those qualities would give her? The answer for the next box was: Feeling complete, full and whole. What would Wholeness give her? She wrote down: Mature wisdom. What would Wisdom give her? She wrote down: The ability to contribute on a much higher level. She was surprised to discover that her relationship goal was actually linked to what she wanted to do through her work as a Coach. She began to sketch out her purpose as being about 'Growing the wisdom to be a source of compassionate support and inspiration.'

Your work is to discover your work and then with all your heart to give yourself to it.

Buddha

Once you have identified your Purpose, or maybe several different purposes, it should be easy for you to create a channel of communication with the part of you that honours and supports this purpose. There is a part of your Heart that has all the resources you need to fulfil your Purpose. Through accessing your Heart, you can tap into wisdom you didn't even know you had. Ideas, inspiration, solutions to problems, inner qualities, and boundless energy can combine to empower you on your path. Whenever you feel stuck, you can receive advice and guidance by connecting with the wisdom of your Heart.

Some people feel this as coming from inside them. Other people meditate, or visualise receiving this guidance from somewhere else. Whatever works for you, is fine. What is important and useful is to have some means to connect with this wisdom whenever you need it. What will help you to remember to listen, take note, and follow the advice that you receive? Here are some easy ways to access your Heart when you need to:

Exercise: Accessing your Heart Wisdom ....

- Take your attention to your Heart or wherever you feel that energy.
- Breathe 10 deep belly breaths while focusing on your Heart.
- Remember times of joy, happiness, compassion, gratitude or love.
- Ask whatever questions you want: seek advice, inspiration, or energy.
- Listen carefully for the answers – be patient and quiet.
- Be willing to commit to following whatever your Heart says.

When you connect with what your Purpose might be, see if you can put it into words. If you can form a phrase or sentence or a poem that sums up your Purpose, it can help you to remember it and stay on track. If you prefer, you could cut out pictures and make a collage that represents your Purpose. Or use any form of creativity to express what this important guiding energy feels like to you. Words are sometimes too small. They diminish the feeling of what your Purpose is. Keep it precious, and you might want to keep it private too. Talking about your Purpose in a mundane way might make it feel less sacred.

Sometimes a symbol or metaphor can help. Long ago, pink roses became a symbol of love and wisdom for me. Whenever I see or smell pink roses, it uplifts me, and my mind immediately accesses peace, innocence, compassion and healing perspectives. So I have pink roses all around my house, and I am always delighted whenever I see roses in gardens, shops, on fabrics or even photos in magazines. The more I can be connected to my resources, the better! So just imagine that you are connecting with your Heart now. If you want, choose a symbol or metaphor to help you, and begin practising tapping into this energy daily.

If you are good at sensing energy, you might already feel that your Purpose does not come from thoughts in your head. People often feel that their Purpose lives somewhere in the centre of their being. In your physical body, your heart has so many neurons, that it actually acts like a separate brain. These neurons have the capability to think for themselves and make decisions separate from the brain in your head. The electromagnetic field of the heart is measured as 5000 times greater than that of the brain. What is interesting is that the type of thinking in your heart often feels quite different from your usual thinking in your head. Try taking your awareness down to your chest right now. Ask yourself how you feel about your Purpose. If you practise accessing your Heart more regularly, it can help guide you to make better decisions.

Your Heart can speak to you easily if you learn how to listen. The messages are always gentle, never judgemental. Its quiet voice is often drowned out by the loud voices in your head. So you need to be still, and direct your attention with care. Ask a question and wait for a true answer. It may come immediately, or through a metaphor, in a dream, or you might just wake up the next morning knowing the answer.

....

How to know it is your Heart talking:

- The message is in alignment with your Purpose
- The voice is usually quiet, sure, strong and peaceful

- The quality is non-judgemental, understanding and wise
- All feelings are honoured, felt, respected and listened to
- It is intuitive, creative and lateral thinking in its solutions
- The essence is always being true to yourself and giving your best
- It only sees Love or situations that require Love for healing
- It feels like an invincible part of you that is always present

Too Good To Be True?

So far we've been taking a totally positive approach to creating the best script for your life. Of course, there will usually be a part of you that objects, doubts, or can't believe this could be of any use at all. This is healthy! In the next chapter, we will start looking at the other side of the story – the less positive scripts you might have been running in your life. We will explore the part of your mind that thinks it is more grounded, realistic, and down to earth. This part of your mind can sometimes be a wet blanket. If yours is pessimistic, over-controlling and critical, it may have been holding you back in many ways. One way it often surfaces is as perfectionism.

Striving for excellence, being diligent and practising regularly are necessary for mastering art, music, dance, and all kinds of sports. We love to watch someone who has perfected the artistry of his work. We admire the expertise and the beauty that results. In fact, the same is true for most professions. It often takes years to develop the proficiency necessary for excellence. When working to perfection flows from following your Heart, your natural gifts flourish. A well-practised flow makes the effort involved in this kind of perfectionism pure joy.

But unhealthy perfectionism can occur when the determination for excellence comes with intolerance. People experience terrible stuck states and extreme frustration when they perceive that what they do isn't perfect enough. Instead of just doing what they love to do, they criticise themselves and get angry. They make comparisons with other people or with an unobtainable ideal that can never be reached. Then they feel miserable.

To a perfectionist, anything less than perfection is failure.

Chuck Spezzano

Sometimes perfectionist people have a war going on inside them. Their internal dialogue constantly criticises everything they do. Unfortunately, when people get really good at criticising themselves, they often generously apply the same to others too. Nothing is ever right. Nothing is ever good enough. All their attention gets focused on what is wrong, or stupid.

A young man in his twenties suffered greatly from perfectionism, which was applied to everything in his life, from his career down to what food he ate. He had suffered from M.E. since he was twelve, and often followed strict diet regimes. He also felt angry all the time, an anger that simmered just below the surface. He became incredibly intolerant when he was driving. Bad customer service made him furious. He felt incredibly frustrated about never having the energy to get his career going. Sometimes he felt like he'd 'crack up', his mind was such a fog that he never seemed to get anywhere.

He believed that to do anything well, you had to learn absolutely everything about that subject first. This led to him starting lots of huge projects, but he never got past the studying stage. He never reached the end, and never got to the point where he could say he succeeded and deserved some free time to relax. Whatever he did manage to do, he judged as not good enough, and often his poor health prevented him from doing things at all. When he applied his perfectionism to his diet, he found he yo-yo'd between being excessively strict, for example by avoiding caffeine, wheat, cigarettes, chocolate, and then completely indulging in all the forbidden things. He'd feel virtuous, in control and great when he was strict. Then he'd rebel, eat all the wrong things and feel terrible both physically and emotionally. Just having a cup of coffee became such a symbol of his indulgence, that it meant that he was not good enough.

When we talked about the perfectionism, he said he didn't feel comfortable at the thought of letting it go. Things just wouldn't be right. Somehow the perfectionism kept him safe, and stopped bad things from happening. His dad, also a perfectionist, was a very tidy, organised man. When he was a boy, his dad had made him put all his toys away – everything had its 'right place'. So he had grown up around a lot of criticism, believing that making a mess was not OK. In order to please his dad, he learned to focus on being perfectly tidy and doing everything just right.

When he explored his past and discovered that the source of his perfectionism went all the way back to childhood, he was surprised. He realised that he must have decided then that it was not safe to be spontaneous and free. But being older and wiser, he could now make a better choice. His Heart gave him some great ways to reframe the old beliefs that were holding him back. He realised that his dad's rules were not necessarily his rules, and those rules might not work for him. Perhaps he could find a way to be spontaneous within the rules that he did consider necessary. He reaffirmed that he was OK just as he is, and didn't have to please everyone. He could have the faith and trust to get 'stuck in', and really feel free to let his creativity out, even if it made a mess!

After our work together, he experienced a distinct shift in his ability to be easier on himself, but there was still an internal battle going on. We discovered there were two internal voices waging war on each other. One was a 'Bully' that governed from his head and used his intellect to make plans and be purposeful. This voice, however, didn't feel safe because the other voice in his chest was like a very, very angry twelve-year-old rebel shouting 'F . . . k you! Nothing works!'

When we explored these two voices more deeply, we discovered that although they had different styles of operation (one wanted safety while the other wanted lots of freedom and experience) they both wanted to experience the magic of life through the senses. They both wanted to relax, connect with everything and beyond to a greater whole. As they realised they both wanted some of the same things, it became easy for them to agree to work together for his benefit.

The young man reflected that all his old rules had been looking outwards – no wonder he had no energy! He had always been driving himself to please other people's standards and to avoid their criticism. From now on, he said, he was going to look inwards and 'live from the inside out'.

Have no fear of perfection, you'll never reach it.

Salvador Dali

If you have a problem with internal voices, locked in a battle of wills, here is an exercise to help you. If you don't have an internal critic, or a voice that casts doubt and cynicism on things that you do, you don't need to do this process. If it ain't broke, don't fix it!

Exercise: Transforming internal critical voices.....................

1. Listen to your internal dialogue and identify any inner critics. If there is more than one voice, work with only one at a time, and complete the process before proceeding to deal with a different voice.
2. Notice where that voice seems to be located in your body or outside your body. Behind you? In front of you? To one side or the other? Move the location of the voice to some distant extremity of your body: your elbow, thumb or big toe . . . or even out in space in front of you. Notice that as it speaks from this new location, that you can listen to what it says more objectively. It may even take on a personality. What does it look like?
3. Presuppose that this voice actually has some positive intent in saying what it says to you. No matter how troublesome it may have been, thank it for all that it has been doing for you over the years and appreciate its intent. Then ask the voice, What is the positive intention behind saying all it says to you? What does it want for you? Listen carefully, and keep asking until you fully understand and appreciate all its positive intentions.
4. Once you know the real intention of this voice, you may discover that the work it does is quite important for you. It may be that you just don't appreciate the style it uses to get your attention. Suggest to this voice that a better way to get your attention and co-operation would be to use attractive, compelling voice tones. Alternatively, change the voice to a friendly cartoon character voice – if it sounds like Mickey Mouse, the message will have a completely different effect on you!

5. Allow the voice – that now sounds so compelling – to move to wherever it considers would be a more comfortable space. How does that feel? What is it like to have this voice as your friend and ally? What becomes easier and more possible?

....

Having done all the exercises so far, are you feeling more positive and excited about your Dream Script? Giving your gifts means that you will be showing up as the person you really came to be. How will you be making a difference in your life, and in other peoples lives? Being guided by your inner Purpose, you will find you have all the strength and courage you need to go for it! You'll be on track with your destiny. Remember these positive resources will always be with you to steady you as you move forward. Think of them as your safety line as you explore what holds you back. If there are wounds that need to be healed, keep your heart steady by remembering the truth of your positive purpose, your gifts and your desirable Dream Script.

Chapter Summary:

Principles:

*You already have all the gifts and resources you need to succeed.
Be kind to yourself.
Avoid the traps of overwhelm and perfectionism.*

Checklist:

1. Identify what gifts you have come to give.
   Identify all your natural talents, qualities, interests or gifts that you already give and will be giving in your ideal script. Use the tick list or just tune into your own unique forms of contribution.
2. What is your Purpose behind the goals you want to achieve?
   Use the Discover Your Purpose exercise for each of your goals. Identify your Purpose and create a special summary statement.
3. Access Your Heart Wisdom.
   Direct your attention to your Heart. Enjoy that energy

and seek its guidance and solutions. Be willing to commit to following its messages. What metaphor might help you connect with your Heart?

4. Transform any internal critical voices.

Follow the process and be sure to honour the positive intent.

4

Appreciating the Present

I was born tomorrow
Today I live
Yesterday killed me.

PARRIZ OWSIA

How does your current life story differ from your Dream Script? Are you happy with the script you are running in your life or would you like to change it? Does it feel like you somehow walked onto the wrong movie set by mistake? Sometimes you might wonder how you ended up in this way of life. Or perhaps you wonder how you can ever get out of this particular script!

How easy is it to change the habits of a lifetime? When you have always behaved a certain way, believed certain things to be true, developed a certain sense of who you are from all that – how can you let go and be different? Many people get stuck in their own comfort zones. They don't like things the way they are, but at least it is the devil they know. Positive change is an unknown territory and therefore risky. You know that habitual behaviours, beliefs and identity are not serving your best interests. Yet you resist making the conscious choices to break through to success. How much of your current script is full of old habits?

Habits form familiar parts of your landscape. Like old friends, they predictably give you the same sort of experience again and again. This sameness lends a certainty and security you can depend on. Who would you be otherwise? How would you have to think differently if you didn't do this anymore? What beliefs might have to change? Appreciate the value of that one important purpose of habit: a comfortable feeling of familiarity. In order to change your script, it may be necessary to risk trying some new behaviours, or changing some old beliefs.

You gain strength, courage and confidence by every experience in which you really stop to look fear in the face. You are able to say to yourself, I lived through this horror. I can take the next thing that comes along.

Eleanor Roosevelt

What Script is Currently Running?

If you were to describe your life, what kind of script do you think it is? A Soap Opera? Drama? Action-packed thriller? Horror movie? Comedy? Documentary? Tragedy? Violent war? What is the general flavour? If your movie was shown on TV, would you be so bored you would change the channel? Do you actually star in your own movie, or are you just a walk-on bit player?

Perhaps you feel pretty happy with your life right now. There may be just a few changes you would like to make. Have a look at a specific area where you feel stuck. Notice what kind of script might be creating that. You may be surprised to discover that you are quite attached to how things are right now. Even though you think you want to do something different, it has served you to have it this way. You might enjoy the drama, even though you yearn for tranquillity. The passion of fights and arguments might be adding a certain zest and energy, even though you want peace. Betrayals, hardships, difficulties may help prove something about you: how strong and clever you are to withstand them, or how much you think you deserve punishment. Failures might be protecting you from having to show up and face even more daunting challenges.

Ask yourself:
- What are the habits or regular problems that occur in your life?
- What do those problems currently add to your life (negatively)?
- What do you yearn for instead?

You need to identify the hidden factors behind what is currently going on in your life. This is the first step to understanding and appreciating the positive points of who you are right now. To honour what is, must precede making changes. Otherwise, internal conflict could arise. How would you know if you had an internal conflict? Have you ever really wanted something but you just couldn't make it happen? Have you ever felt like something sabotaged your best plans and good intentions? Do you have a part inside that doesn't feel heard, recognised, appreciated or respected? Indeed, you may be well aware that you have a part you don't like very much at all. If you locate one side of an inner conflict, it presumes the existence of its opposite.

Exercise: Identify your current script......................................

1. Identify what general type of script is currently running. What is the plot?
2. What are the common themes that are running in your movie? Here are some common themes that might be lurking:

Blaming, judging, being right	**Victim**
Trapped, stuck, controlled	**Held back**
Competition, warfare, power struggle.............	**Revenge**
Losing, defeated, hopeless	**Failure**
Disappointment, hurt, grief	**Heartbreak**
Lost, separate, invisible...............................	**Abandonment**
Cheating, infidelity, jealousy	**Betrayal**
Not good enough, worthless..........................	**Rejection**
Giving up, frustration, no hope.....................	**Depression**
Accidents, disability, disease	**Illness**
Unworthy, low self esteem, helpless...............	**Inadequacy**
Giving too much, dependent...........................	**Sacrifice**
Being at fault, bad, punished........................	**Guilt**
Dissociated, unfeeling, inertia	**Boredom**
Indulgence, temptation, out of control............	**Addiction**
Holding on, demands, power struggle............	**Control**

3. What does playing this role cause you to feel? Are there any feelings of apathy, grief, fear, lust, anger, sadness, guilt or pride? Any other feelings?
4. When did you first notice you had this kind of script running? Have there been frequent reruns of the same kind of story?

5. What purpose did this script serve? What did it allow you to avoid? In what way did it help you to hide, or avoid giving some gift?
6. How would this story continue? How would you expect it to unfold? If nothing changes, where will you be in five years time? Ten years time?
7. What are the challenges or problems occurring in this script? List them.
8. How much would you like to change this script? (Score 1–10)

Example: One client was running a heartbreak/betrayal/rejection script with a plot that ran a series of tragic love affairs that never ended well. The theme was always the same: unrequited love that ended in total rejection, leaving the heroine feeling worthless. The feelings usually started with falling in love (lust), often involved jealousy and then ended with bags of anger and sadness, leading to hopeless depression and grief. At first, she thought it started with her early love affairs, but after thinking it over carefully, she realised that she had felt the same feelings with her father, even when she was a young girl. The purpose behind this script was harder to fathom, but it seemed to be about holding herself back. She spent so much time focusing on these relationships and recovering from the heartbreaks, that she had little energy left to develop her career. So she successfully avoided giving most of her talents and gifts. This allowed her to feel safe. If the series continued, there would be more and more rejections until she would probably finally give up and consider herself totally worthless and unlovable. The challenges in this particular script were about learning how to love herself.

Before you can create your Dream Script in your life, it is essential to understand, appreciate and honour your current script. Your current script requires lots of compassion. There is always some purpose or message hidden behind the action. The intention behind what is happening may or may not seem totally positive at first. But if you continue to explore the repercussions of its purpose, you will most likely discover the reasoning that led to the unusual outcomes that you experienced as your current script.

There is a Positive Intention Behind Every Behaviour

Does it sound strange to think that there is a positive intention behind every behaviour? First consider who has the intention. The positive intention will usually serve the person doing the action, not necessarily anyone else. Very few people actually set out to do harm. They are usually protecting themselves or trying to get something they want. Often they don't realise the effect it might have on others.

When thinking about your current script, be curious about what hidden intention it could have. It may not be serving what you want (consciously), but it may be doing a good job satisfying some hidden needs. Notice that every behaviour is an attempt to get something or avoid something. When you are trying to avoid something, that really means you want something else instead. Be curious to discover what that could be. Maybe you already know that positive intention. Some people prefer to deny that there could be any such intention. Things like getting ill so that you can't perform, could be about protecting you from fear of failure or being exposed as a fraud.

Your hidden intentions govern your behaviour subconsciously. Then every thought, every feeling, and every action starts a snowball of subsequent thoughts and actions. Whatever is happening in your life right now, could only be that way because of previous thoughts, decisions, feelings, beliefs and actions. It is rather like programming a computer: if you put garbage in, you get garbage out. Therefore it helps to know what those hidden intentions might be. Then you have choice about changing them. If you are not aware of your hidden positive intentions, how could you choose differently?

Your mind started acquiring programmes long before you had the wisdom to choose. Your true inner self may have always known your purpose, but this became hidden underneath less useful programmes. No matter how bad the input though, there was always some payoff, some reason for originally accepting those programmes. You need to find out what that was. Then you can find other ways to satisfy that hidden intention or let it go. Your current script just has bad habits. No matter how ingrained the behaviour, the beliefs, or how much your old script may have held you back, you can change anything you want by re-writing your script.

Discovering a Hidden Purpose

Discovering the hidden purpose behind your current script requires good detective work. This story about a client in an outraged state shows how complex the reasoning can be. John had previously worked through issues to do with anger, but he still found himself in the same habit, running the same old victim script. His internal anger was spoiling for a fight, looking for any suitable target.

Listening to the long list of complaints that stretched from his present all the way back to his childhood, it was clear that his stories were well worn and familiar: old grievances, hurts, wounds, and slights. His favourite one was a terrible story of injustice. When he was a little boy, he had a bad habit of leaving his treasured bicycle lying in the driveway. His father found this extremely annoying when he came home to park his car and told him many times to put it away properly. Of course, he forgot. Unfortunately, this time his father came home, became enraged and ran over the bicycle on purpose, just to teach his son a lesson. To make it worse, the bicycle was never replaced. Instead of learning the lesson of tidiness and consideration, however, this little four-year-old boy learned how to feel like a powerless victim. With repeated incidents like this, he also learned how to justify his victim status with evidence and right-eous indignation. It become such a strong habit he said, 'I don't know what to do with myself unless I perceive struggle and hardship to complain about.'

What could possibly be the positive benefit for him in repeating his journey down this angry street, complaining and struggling? Curiously, whenever he thought about his potential, his capabilities or what he really wanted to do with his life, an internal voice derided him for being arrogant and presumptuous. Then he would go into battle against this internal foe. Not surprisingly, this internal voice sounded a lot like his father. He said his father had not been 'man enough' to allow him to grow up, but instead pushed him down with criticism, and crushed his dreams. As a boy, he lived in fear of his father, learning to avoid his wrath. He thought his survival depended on keeping everyone happy. But his father's injustice outraged him. As he held the anger inside his body, it made him feel more alive. It was as though the anger gave him confirmation of his existence – it made his nerves tingle!

We explored what this angry part really wanted for him. It was complicated! Whenever he fell victim to someone's bad behaviour, he felt sorry for himself. This led to a feeling of self-righteousness, where he was ultimately right, and everyone else was wrong. He got so much satisfaction from proving how ultimately right he was, he began to think the rest of the whole world was wrong and against him; a negative conspiracy theory. His righteousness extended to proving God wrong for having created the world to be so horrible. He loved being able to say, 'I told you so!' to God. Then, having won his fight with God, he felt the peace of feeling totally superior. At last, he felt everyone would notice him, look up to him, and value him for his greatness. He would be able to have everything he wanted. He'd get all his needs met, living life to the full. Here he imagined he could feel content, happy, fulfilled with nothing to prove anymore. Unfortunately, he didn't get to that place very often, nor could he stay there very long.

When he felt calm and objective, he was able to connect with his Heart's purpose of contentment. Then he could think more compassionately about all the different stories that had created his angry script. Remembering his inner gifts of fulfilment and happiness gave him the strength to access deeper inner truth and his innate value. In this good state, it was easier to understand and forgive both his own mistakes and those of others. He realised he had never forgiven himself for not standing up to his father.

In fact, he had made his whole life about winning the competition to be better than his dad. Yet, even as a young boy, he intuitively knew he was already smarter than his dad. Oddly enough, a part of him believed that being totally successful would diminish and demolish his father. So he held himself back, confused between trying to win his father's love by staying small and competing with him at the same time. Deep down, he loved his dad. He gradually realised that the greatest gift he could give his father would be his success, as well as gratitude for teaching him how to work hard.

Although there were contexts at work where using his old anger script might still be useful, he began to find it much easier to choose compassion. He started seeing his father with forgiveness and understanding. He found he was able to access his Heart much more easily.

All the world's a stage,
And all the men and women merely players:
They have their exits and their entrances;
And one man in his time plays many parts.

William Shakespeare

Who is Starring in Your Current Movie Script?

Have you ever noticed that you sometimes play very different roles in your life? Some people think this is just passing moods. People even say, 'I just wasn't myself that day' or 'I don't know what came over me!' Maybe you've had the experience of saying things you really regret later on, or doing things that make you cringe to remember them. What is happening? Who is in control of your mouth? What was it that made you do that?

What makes this even more puzzling is that sometimes you can justify everything you do, and sometimes you can't. But you try to convince yourself and others that you have the best reasons, the best intentions, the most intellectual rationale for whatever you do. But somehow it doesn't match with what other parts of you think and feel. Even worse, the results and the aftermath are not really what you wanted at all. Oops.

Maybe you've noticed this happen in people around you: a person can predictably behave one way, and then totally contradict themselves in the next moment. Although you could put it down to moods, these roles are difficult to deal with. Each role has different attitudes, different values and different desired outcomes. Different circumstances trigger each role to think it is their cue to come on stage. Each role also has a history dating back to a time when it was useful to behave the way it does. Hence, the old issues of the past tend to re-surface and become re-enacted. Have you ever noticed how your life tends to repeat certain types of experiences again and again?

Are you aware of old unresolved issues, conflicts or wounds that were left unhealed in the past? Each of these created a role as a coping mechanism. The different behaviours of each role fulfil hidden needs and intentions. They are doing their best to resolve or hide the old problems. Until the original issues can be understood with compassion, the conflicts between the differing roles can pull you apart, interfere with your true purpose and obstruct your Dream Script path and destiny. What happened to the man in the following story is not so uncommon.

> *There is no conflict that does not entail*
> *The single, simple question, 'What am I?'*
>
> A Course in Miracles

A marriage of thirteen years was hitting difficulties. The wife told the husband she just couldn't live with him anymore and she wanted a divorce. No matter how he tried to convince himself that this was a welcome opportunity, the truth was that he really didn't want a divorce or to be parted from his kids. With great *Sadness*, he told me how much he loved his wife and how precious she was to him, and what a happy home they had. His future now looked so bleak, he contemplated suicide.

His father had ruled his childhood like an absolute dictator. His mother had been very manipulative, needy, and clinging. No matter what he did, it was never good enough for his father, and never enough to satisfy his mother. His one act of defiance was to choose a wife who was totally unacceptable to both his parents. What he loved about his wife most was that she imposed no rules, and that she nurtured him and met his needs. Now with the impending divorce, he felt his whole life was complete *Desolation*.

Although his wife had made a good job of rescuing him, she had begun to resent his neediness. She felt suffocated by him. She complained that he was super critical, that he always knew better, and he was a bully. He admitted that he often told her and the children how to do things, like the plates had to be rinsed before being put in the dishwasher, and lights had to be turned out if you left a room. He had 'reasonable' rules for just about everything and was convinced his way was usually 'right'. He was uncompromising in imposing his rules. Not surprisingly, his wife found it intolerable to be on the receiving end of this every day.

It was as if he had become a combination of all the bad qualities that he hated so much in his own parents, becoming both *Needy* and a dictator. He was appalled to realise the effect it had, and resolved immediately to give up his need to be right, and change his critical correcting behaviour. Within only a few days, his wife and kids were really enjoying the new, laid-back, easy-going dad, and some progress was made towards a reconciliation.

But by his next visit, he was very *Angry* that his improvements had not stopped the divorce proceedings. He was like a different person expressing nothing but negative judgements about his wife. His criticism, indignation, and rage seemed boundless. He questioned whether he really loved his wife, or whether such a thing as love existed! Life seemed without purpose or meaning, as his intellectual skills were now focused entirely on justifying his anger. He found it hard to switch out of *Mr Angry* as his mind was so preoccupied with all the reasons and justifications for his behaviour.

After we did a process to release his anger, much to his surprise, he suddenly remembered how much he really loved his wife and tears fell from his eyes. I drew his attention to how his whole demeanour vacillated from being *Mr Sad* and *Desolate*, to *Mr Needy*, to *Mr Angry*, to *Mr Loving*. It was as if he was playing multiple roles, each with different objectives, different values and different feelings. Sometimes he even brought in a *Mr Demon* role that only wanted complete devastation and destruction!

I asked him which of these roles was the real him? And if he were to follow the path each one of them directed, which one would help him have what he truly wanted – his wife and happy family back? Appealing to his love of logic, I asked him to imagine what sort of results *Mr Sad* and *Desolate* would reap? What would happen if *Mr Needy* operated 100 per cent of the time? Where would he end up if *Mr Angry* continued? What would it be like if he could be *Mr Loving*?

It was obvious that no matter how tempting it was to follow the other paths, to indulge in the feeling of being right, or to punish everyone for not meeting his needs, the only path that made any sense, the only path that felt true was the *Loving* one. It was also the only path that could possibly help to heal his marriage. But he objected that it was not so easy to just 'choose' to be loving! It might not be easy, but who is in control of your thoughts and feelings if you are not? Who writes your script? Who directs your life if you don't? You must begin with making that essential choice of who you truly want to be, and then allow that to guide your thoughts, your words and your actions.

Making that choice becomes easier after you learn how to heal some of the old issues from your past. When the old wounds are healed they no longer trigger you. But find out first what roles you are currently acting in your current life script.

Who are you choosing to be in the script you are running right now? There may be several roles that you play. First it helps to get acquainted with each different role, how it feels and what it wants for you. You may be aware of only one main role, but if you feel resistance to that, there must be at least two.

Exercise: What roles are you playing in your current script?

1. Identify what role(s) you are aware of playing in your current script. Notice if there are any feelings connected with that. Imagine what this role might say and write it down.
   Example: One client was playing a helpless victim role. She noticed she had a lot of silent complaints constantly running through her head. She wrote them all down and realised she was really very angry about many things, but was not expressing that anger openly because another part of her thought she didn't have the right to, people wouldn't think she was nice, or she wouldn't be safe if she did.
2. If you find there is a battle going on inside your head, separate the different roles and carefully write down what

each of them thinks. Keep a separate list for each one.
Example: This same client then wrote down all the things the angry voice wanted and all the things the fearful voice was afraid of.

3. Working with only one list at a time, determine: what is the objective and intention of each role?
Example: Her angry voice was actually trying to protect her, and stand up for herself and what she considered to be important. While the fearful voice was ringing alarm bells about how she could possibly be hurt again like she had been in the past. It wanted safety.

4. What does each role really want for you by behaving as it does? Repeat that question until you have discovered the highest intentions. Sometimes, there might be some negative answers. If you discover a really angry or hopeless role that wants to die, find out what it thinks death would give you. Usually there is a belief that death would bring peace or some other positive resolution. Write down all the objectives.
Example: Her victim role wanted her to avoid feeling guilty by blaming everyone else as the bad guys. Then she could feel innocent and hard done by, justifying all the angry complaining. Being a victim really meant that she was powerless to change things, and was hoping to be rescued and taken care of. Believing herself to be powerless was really a form of self-attack, a way to deny her true inner power and ability to choose. It meant she didn't have to show up, or put out any effort to change herself or the situations she complained about. This was hiding a deeper fear that she wasn't good enough or smart enough. By avoiding all responsibility, she wouldn't be found lacking. This gave her a form of protection and security.

5. Look over the answers objectively and compassionately to gain more understanding of what each part might be trying to positively gain for you. Don't stop until you have discovered all the positive gains.

6. With regard to what you want in your life right now, which part is most likely to be helpful? Which one is the true star of your show? It is your choice. (Reminder: it is usually advisable to ask your Heart to answer this question, not your head.)

> Example: *She discovered another part of her that realised she was not a victim. This part had courage and believed she was OK the way she is. Although she was not used to listening to this part, she was willing to choose this one to star in her Dream Script.*

Small Details Reveal Clues

If you are having difficulty discovering the hidden dynamics of your script, or you are coaching someone else, sometimes it helps to pay attention to the small details of what is being communicated. Remember that communication is not just the words being said. The tone of voice, the speed and emphasis give you much of the meaning. People also communicate through how they dress, their posture, what gestures they make and how they behave. It is amusing to notice that even the tiny metaphors of jewellery can reveal a message. From the overall big picture down to the smallest details there will be clues about the roles being played to help you discover what is going on. Sometimes it is also necessary to listen to what is not being said. What is being left out, forgotten, or denied can speak volumes. You may need to look at what is missing from the picture or what doesn't add up. Reading between the lines will help you spot the areas that are out of the person's awareness.

A good example of this was given by an attractive client who arrived a bit late for her appointment. In fact, she told me she had arrived so early, she had decided to go for a walk in the park, and then got lost! I noticed she had her shirt on backwards, she had her watch on upside-down, and she was wearing little earrings made of interwoven knots. Before she spoke, I was already wondering about how confused she might be, what she might be looking back at, and how she was tied up in knots. She told me that although her career was going just great, she didn't feel she knew what she really wanted to do. After several relationship failures, she had become dissatisfied with everything. Although she tried to see all events as positive opportunities for change, she often felt very unfocused.

Ever since she could remember she had always been the 'responsible one' in her family. People thought she was the eldest child, even though she had an older sister and younger brother. Her father had always treated her as an equal. Although he had been an extremely difficult person to get along with, she greatly missed the deep sense of security and safety that he had provided so well. Since his death, she suspected that she had been hoping to re-create that security in many of her relationships.

She admitted that most of her relationships had been disastrous – in fact she called them 'lucky escapes'! None of them had ever worked out and for a long time she simply didn't have any close relationships. I asked her how much she was still 'holding on' to her father? She said 80 per cent. Then we worked out how much she was also still 'holding on' to five of the major relationships that hadn't worked out – it added up to another 80 per cent. So her energy was 160 per cent still attached to these past relationships. No wonder she did not attract a new partner. She really was tied up in knots.

Whenever a relationship failed, no matter who decided to end it, she felt like a failure. Despite reading self-help books, attending relationship seminars and seeing therapists, she didn't feel that she was making any progress. The same patterns tended to repeat themselves, and she just ended up feeling depressed. Sometimes her sense of failure was so intense that her inner critic would tell her, 'You are not good enough to live.'

We explored this idea of 'not being good enough'. She said she felt like she always had to work twice as hard as everyone else, just to be acceptable. No matter how well she performed, it was never good enough. She had very low self-worth, and found it difficult to express her thoughts and needs. It felt like she didn't deserve to be loved. She simply was not important enough.

Tracing this feeling back to her childhood, she remembered many fights with her older sister. Her sister had never been happy to have the competition of a younger child around. She would often hit her until she started crying. Then one or both parents would intervene and punish both girls for misbehaving. Somehow this resulted in a mistaken belief that she was guilty, just for being alive. Later when her brother was born, the attention she used to receive as the youngest child was suddenly focused on the baby. Her belief in her lack of worth solidified. She must have decided to spend the rest of her life trying to pay this imaginary guilty debt.

I reminded her to connect with her Heart, and remember her true giftedness. The guidance from her Heart helped. She reframed the mistake that she could be anything but lovable and worthy. She realised how loved she was, and how she could protect herself. In fact, everything was just fine. She was OK and other people were OK too. She acknowledged that it was important and precious to feel whatever her feelings were, but it was better not to linger in negative feelings. She decided to stop carrying this experience around with her. She was ready to move on and reach out to others, knowing that she is good enough. Just being who she is, is enough.

Next she was ready to let go of her attachments to her father and previous relationships. Her energy felt clear and open. Able to move forward at last, she focused her attention on what criteria she would really like in her true life partner. She began to create her new Dream Script.

> *Love will enter immediately into any mind that truly wants it, but it must want it truly.*
>
> *A Course in Miracles*

Hidden Fears

Often there are deep feelings underneath the roles you play in your current life script. Just like you discovered that your Dream Script may aspire to fulfil desires to be loved, approved of, in control and safe, the story you tell with your current life script can reveal not only hidden agendas, intentions and purposes but also hidden fears. There are three basic channels of fear that seem to breed all of the other negative feelings. In their most extreme form they are:

Hopelessness: I'll never be loved, never get what I want
Helplessness: I'm out of control, can't change anything
Worthlessness: I'm not good enough, don't deserve to live

In milder forms, they might be harder to recognise, but if you were to exaggerate whatever feeling is associated with your current script, you will probably discover that it relates to one or two of these basic fears. Sometimes all three will combine to create a complicated cocktail of negative feelings. At this point just be curious about which fears occur with most regularity. Please remember to stay connected to your Heart, your giftedness, and your purpose in order to maintain your balance. Old habits can be seductive.

Once you recognise that your fears follow one of these three channels, however, it will become easier to choose a different path. With practice, you'll be able to recognise more quickly what triggers you and tempts you to re-run an old script again. 'Oh, there you go again, running the "no one loves you", or "you're not good enough", or "nothing will ever change" script!' After you've learned how to transform these mistakes in your thinking, you will never be fooled into thinking they could be true again.

It's Your Choice: You can be Right, or Happy.

Although you may think you have lots of evidence to prove one of these negative beliefs, ultimately it boils down to a choice you have to make for yourself. You can choose useful beliefs that reframe old patterns of thinking and leave you feeling resourceful, strong, loving, happy and able to give your best. Or you can continue to believe unhelpful, fearful, negative ideas that prove how right you are to feel helpless, hopeless or worthless.

Every decision is a choice between love and fear.
A Course in Miracles

Worthlessness

Consider worthlessness objectively. Can you think of anyone who isn't good enough, or doesn't deserve to live? No matter how negatively you might judge someone or something, ultimately there is some use, some purpose there. Even a piece of rubbish on the street is a banquet to the insects that thrive on it. There probably isn't anything in the universe that doesn't have some positive purpose for existing.

Most people would at least begrudgingly admit that every human life is precious, and every person is worthy no matter how poor, sick, or unfortunate. Yet many of those same people choose to view themselves as unworthy because they focus on making comparisons to some imagined ideal. This form of self-judgement actually sets them apart, makes them more special than everyone else on earth. 'Everyone else is worthy, but not me' they say. Can this be the truth?

If you ask your Heart for a true evaluation of your worth, you will get a very different answer. If you access your deeper inner self, you will realise that you are just as deserving as anyone else. If you think about it logically, the very fact that you are alive must be evidence in favour of your worth. The universe doesn't create junk. If the universe is a hologram, then you must be a very important corner of that hologram. Without you, the universe would not be complete. You can choose to remember your true worth instead of making comparisons and judgements that you are not good enough. You are good enough and there is always room for improvement!

Hopelessness

Hopelessness comes from imagining that things will never work out. You will never achieve your dreams, or never be loved the way you've always wanted. Why would you want to imagine a future like that? Maybe things haven't worked out in the past, but you never know what is around the next corner. You cannot predict what wonderful things could happen. It may not be exactly what you planned or hoped for, but whatever surprises occur could be a new adventure of discovery and growth.

If you are attached to a certain outcome, or to having a particular person to love, then it is easy to feel that your hopes have been dashed when things don't work out. However, most people have had experiences that didn't work out, and later on that turned out to be a blessing in disguise. They thanked their lucky stars that they didn't get what they thought they wanted. If your life isn't happening according to your plans, maybe you've got the wrong plans! If it hasn't happened, maybe it wasn't meant to happen. Maybe there's something better and more appropriate for you.

It is much more useful to have an attitude of curiosity and a willingness to enjoy the adventures that your life constantly offers you. If you let go of your attachment to how you think things should be, you might begin to notice how wonderful things are. You might become more aware of little opportunities that could open up whole new avenues of possibility and happiness. What if hopeless feelings are just a signal that it is time for you to create a new script? Wouldn't it be more useful to give your best regardless of whether or not your plans worked out? Then, no matter what happened, you could just enjoy the adventure.

Helplessness

Whether you feel out of control or whether you are an obsessive control freak, you may be frightened of being helpless. When you feel you can't change anything because you are a victim of other people's decisions, or actions, it is tempting to feel helpless and give away your power. Maybe you feel like a victim of fate, that the universe is conspiring against you. Thinking like this could make you feel small, helpless, fearful and unable to give your best.

Conversely, the horror of not being able to control everything important to your survival can make you behave like a tyrant. You might feel you need to dictate every detail and manipulate every event so that you can feel secure. But holding on so tightly and forcing your will, is fear-based behaviour that can obstruct the creative unfolding process of your life.

Issues about being in control are central to your sense of identity. Whether you behave like a helpless victim or a thundering tyrant, neither role reveals your true identity. Who you are may have nothing to do with how much control you have over the events in your life. What would your Heart say about how powerful you are? What is the truth about whether or not you manage to control everything in your life? What is important about your survival? Are you just this bag of bones and flesh, or are you much more than that? What is your true identity?

If you could remember who you truly are, how incredible, magnificent, unique, gifted, innocent, joyful, loving and powerful you are, control would no longer be an issue. When you realise that you have actually asked for things to be the way they are, consciously or subconsciously, you will appreciate how creative your thoughts are. Wouldn't it be more useful to flow with the current of your life, rather than fight against it? Learning to listen to your inner guidance and respond to events could help you find a true source of happiness rather than struggling to be in control.

Ask your Heart:
- Who am I? What is my true identity? What is my worth?
- What is great about the events that are happening?
- What opportunities might be opening up for me right now?
- How much power do I have?
- How could I best respond to what is happening right now?

For a more detailed, complete assessment of what stands in your way of creating your Dream Script, here is an amazing exercise that will provide you with a road map to find out what needs to be healed in order to find your way to happiness and manifest your Dream Script coming true.

Exercise: Healing what holds you back

Use a large sheet of paper for this exercise:

1. Write a one sentence description of your Dream Script in the grey box, or put in one of your important goals.
2. Ask yourself what stops you from having that right now? When you come up with an answer, put it in one of the top limitation boxes. Keep asking what stops you until you have all the limitations that get in the way. (You can have as many boxes as you like going across the page.)
3. Pick one of the limitations, and concentrate on only that box. Ask yourself, what would you like to have instead of that limitation? Put this in the new outcome box directly below the limitation.
4. Referring to what you just wrote, ask yourself what stops you

from having this new outcome? Put this in a limitation box below the new outcome.

5. Ask what you would like to have instead of this limitation, and put the answer in a box below. You should be creating a vertical column of boxes alternating limitations with new outcomes. Keep repeating the two questions until you reach a point where what is in the last box is a positive behaviour that is possible for you to take action on right away.

Keep repeating the two alternate questions until you reach a new outcome in each column that is easily achievable or links to another column.

OUTCOME: What do you want in your script?

⬇

What stops you?	What else stops you?	And what else stops you?

⬇   ⬇   ⬇

LIMITATION	LIMITATION	LIMITATION

⬇   ⬇   ⬇

What do you want instead? (Do one column at a time)

⬇   ⬇   ⬇

NEW OUTCOME	NEW OUTCOME	NEW OUTCOME

Example:

I want to be a successful Coach

| What stops you? | What else stops you? | And what else stops you? |

  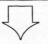

| *Need skills* | *No clients* | *Lack confidence* |

  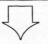

What do you want instead? (Do one column at a time)

| *Recognised training* | *Join network / referrals* | *Skills & expertise* |

| What stops you? | What stops you? | What stops you? |

 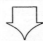

| *Lack funding* | *Lack confidence* | *Need practice* |

What do you want instead? (Do one column at a time)

| *Research loans, & save* | | *Work with friends* |

When you have completed this exercise, you should have gained clarity about precisely which areas require some healing and where new resources are needed. You may find that one column of limitations is linked to another. The ideal outcome for this exercise is that you now have several tasks at the bottom of the page. They should give you ideas about actions you can begin right now. You can start working towards making your Dream Script a reality. These should be things you know you can do, and they may even bring a smile to your face. In the next chapter you will find more information about dealing with issues that require healing.

> *The main fact of life for me is love or its absence.*
> *Whether life is worth living depends on whether there is*
> *love in life.*
>
> R. D. Laing

Guilt

Guilt is a difficult mixture of worthlessness, hopelessness and helplessness. It deserves a special mention because it is often so hard to identify, yet it is so effective at keeping people stuck. Often when there is guilt, there is indebtedness as well, which keeps the pattern running indefinitely.

Feeling that you do not deserve to have a wonderful life, or thinking your Dream Script is impossible, usually indicates that you feel guilty about something. Do you feel totally innocent and deserving of every good thing? If you do, you probably already have everything you want. When you don't allow yourself to receive everything you want, consider it to be a measure of how much guilt you unconsciously store. How would you be able to tell if you are carrying unconscious levels of guilt? Look at areas of your life where you have withdrawn your energy, places where you are hiding and not showing up. You might call it shyness. You might have all kinds of excuses about why you are hiding. Look deeper. What are you afraid people might find out about you?

Guilt is a strange emotion. It is harder to recognise than other emotions, since it doesn't usually display distinct physical qualities.

With sadness, you cry; with anger, you turn red, feel hot, shout; with fear, you tremble and go cold; but with guilt? Everyone hates to feel that something is their fault. Some people go to amazing lengths to avoid guilt by pinning the blame on someone else. In families, one person often ends up being the scapegoat and taking all the guilt. It is so much easier to blame someone else than feel guilty oneself.

When you have guilt, at some level you feel you are bad, and you fear that your badness might show, so you create elaborate strategies of hiding. Withdrawing, not showing up, not succeeding, and being ingratiating are all common signs of guilt. A more deceptive way to hide guilt is to attack, bully, and dominate because you secretly feel you lack power, and fear being found out. Guilt is usually behind the feeling that you are a fraud. But the strangest thing is that there is often no reason to feel guilty in the first place! It is a mistake.

Ask yourself:
- Does a part of me feel that I don't deserve to have my Dream Script?
- Where do I hold myself back, hide, not show up or feel shy?
- What do I fear people might find out about me?

If you are not aware of anything to feel guilty about consciously, look at where you try to place blame on someone else. What you judge in other people often reflects what you are blind to see in yourself. If only they were different! It is their fault! They are doing something bad. Look deeper: how and where are you doing something very similar – possibly in the way you treat yourself? Or think about times other people have tried to make you feel guilty and bad. Notice that if they had said, 'you shouldn't have robbed that bank', you would shrug it off because it wouldn't have any sting. But the accusations that stick, fester because there is some guilt present acting as the glue. Those are the places where you believe you are truly guilty in some way.

When did you start to feel guilty? Was there a specific event? Was there a pattern in your family – did you always think everything was your fault somehow? Many children make this mistake. If you can, identify the earliest event and gather the facts. When guilt runs deep, it usually carries feelings of helplessness, hopelessness and worthlessness.

If you are finding this hard to relate to, perhaps this story about a beautiful young personal assistant will make it clear. Despite her beauty, she felt very guilty and very distressed without knowing why. She hated being a PA because she spent all her time and energy making someone else's life more important than her own. Despite always being a high achiever, she had extremely low self-esteem. Despite being gorgeous, she had never had a fulfilling relationship. She felt that she was not pretty enough, not thin enough, not intelligent enough – just not worthy enough to be loved. So she spent all her time running around after other people, taking care of everyone's needs and believing the purpose of her life was to make others' lives better. She also believed that a sense of worth and deserving could only come from hard work. If things came easily, they were not deserved and of no importance. Not surprisingly, she was a hard taskmaster on herself, always striving to achieve more, but equally scared of taking risks or doing what she really wanted.

When did she stop believing that she was worth anything? Why did she feel she didn't even exist? Why did she decide to be everyone's caretaker? She traced the feeling back to the time when she was six years old, when her little brother was born. There was a significant moment when the whole family was gathered in the living room, her parents, grandparents, her sister and herself, all admiring the new baby boy. As she ran between them all, she realised that everything had changed. She had gone from being the precious youngest child, getting all the attention, to just being the second daughter, worthy of none. The family, for many generations, had revered having sons. To make matters worse, her mother's first child had been a son who died after birth. Consequently, this new baby boy was now the focus of excessive care and attention.

The little girl struggled to find some way to be special again. She mistakenly decided that she had done something wrong, and she wasn't good enough, therefore, she was being punished. She decided to be the 'action kid': if something needed doing, she'd do it! She thought if she did things very well, they'd love her again. Since she was naturally very capable, this led to learning lots of ways to help people and to be an achiever. Sadly though, the family adopted an attitude that because she was so good at everything, she didn't require as much attention as the other two children. So when she got even less attention, she tried even harder to please, and even tried to win their love by making herself small. She cut off all her hair to look less pretty and acted more like a tomboy.

Feeling that all her efforts to get a sense of value from others had failed, she had stopped believing she was worth anything. She had stopped looking after herself. She was afraid to be successful, attractive or feminine. Hence she ended up working as a PA despite all her qualifications. She had forgotten who she was. Slowly she began to realise that all her caring had been a false kind of giving, in order to get love and attention. Her whole life had been a 'sacrifice script', a form of counterfeit giving.

Working with the origin of her decision to become everyone's carer at six years old, she accessed her Heart for guidance. She then realised that she was lovable and had always been loved, despite the displacement of attention. It was OK to just be who she is. She didn't have to do things to be loved. Instead of feeling desperate, she knew that she really was being seen and heard. She began to feel that she deserved love, and that she could even begin to love herself.

Then she confessed that she didn't really know what it meant to love herself, so, for homework, she agreed to think about and write down all the different ways she could love herself. Not just about treating herself with bubble baths and her favourite foods, but all the different ways she could begin to treat herself with respect, stand up for what she valued, and be more kind and forgiving about any mistakes she might make. As she began to see herself as innocent, her guilt evaporated.

The supreme happiness of life is the conviction that we are loved, loved for ourselves, or rather, loved in spite of ourselves.

Victor Hugo

How well do you treat yourself with love?
- Do you take good care of yourself? Your health? Your body?
- How easy is it for you to treat yourself without feeling guilty?
- How many ways could you stand up for what is true for you?
- How well are you living your Purpose?
- Do you remember to appreciate all the things you do well?
- Are you kind and forgiving when you make a mistake?
- What are other ways you love yourself?

What if you DO have reason to feel guilty? What if you really have done something bad? Some people believe that they must hold onto the guilt forever, just because they have made a mistake. People can be very hard on themselves. If you never let yourself off the hook, then the old guilt breeds more bad behaviour. What you focus on is what you get! Subconscious guilt will guide your awareness, your thoughts, intentions, and your behaviour. Even if you are thinking 'I must not think of guilt, I must not think of that bad thing I did . . .' your mind is making pictures of guilt. Like a magnet, those negative thoughts will attract more negative feelings and behaviour.

The true purpose of guilt is for you to learn the lesson, not build a monument to the mistake. Once you realise your mistake, have the wisdom to make a better choice and do things differently. Then commit to never doing that again. It is time to move on, let go of the guilt, and let go of the past. The future does not have to look like the past. Holding on to what has happened in the past may just be an excuse to hide your fear of taking a step forward into your Dream Script. Forgive yourself for past mistakes and re-connect with the truth of your basic innocence once again.

Having identified what kind of script you have been running, what roles you have been playing, what purpose your current script has, and what the hidden intentions and needs are behind the scenes, you are now ready to begin the transformation part of the process. Remember to stay connected to your Heart, your gifts and your true Purpose so that you can stay balanced. Sometimes old issues and problems try to tempt you back into old feelings and behaviours. Resist this! It cannot be true for you. There's got to be a better way. In the next two chapters you will learn how to heal what has held you back.

Chapter Summary
Principles:
Behind every behaviour is a positive intention
You choose who directs your script
You can re-connect with your innocence

Checklist:
1. What is the current script that is running in your life?
   a. Identify what kind of script you are running
   b. What feelings are associated with that?
2. When did you start running this script? Has it been re-run many times?
   a. What purpose does your current script serve?
   b. How would this story continue and unfold?
   c. What challenges or problems does this script reveal?
3. Who is starring in your script – do you play more than one role?
   a. Notice any internal conflicts
   b. What is the purpose or positive intention of each role? What does each want for you?
   c. Which one is most likely to be helpful? Which one is the true star of your story?
4. What hidden fears might be behind these intentions – what are the hidden needs?
   a. Hopelessness
   b. Helplessness
   c. Worthlessness
5. What stops you from having your Dream Script?
   a. Use the Healing what holds you back exercise.
   b. Discover what limits you.
   c. Decide what you want instead.
6. Assess how much unconscious guilt might be hiding behind some of your intentions and behaviours.
   a. Choose to re-connect with your Heart.
   b. Commit to learning the lesson.
   c. Move on.

5

Honouring Hidden Intentions

Nothing but your own thoughts can hamper your progress.

A COURSE IN MIRACLES

If what you focus on is what you get, then why doesn't everyone have everything they want? It must be because they are focusing on something different from what they think they want. Your current life script follows your subconscious stories more than your conscious desires. Once upon a time, you made decisions about what was happening in your life. The stories that emerged from the old needs that didn't get fulfilled, accumulated and formed your current script. Whatever is happening in your current life script therefore serves some old purpose. You could go as far as to say that your subconscious chooses how your life is right now. From the major events down to the smallest details, your script continues to try to heal the old needs.

Sometimes your script might resemble childhood fairy tales, legends, comic books, movies or something from history. Often these types of stories hide old heartbreaks, failures or guilt from the past. There might have been a traumatic event that you felt you didn't handle very well. So in your story you attempt to become the heroic character who has the strength, skills, or courage to succeed where you once failed. By playing out this role on an unconscious level, you hope to rectify the past and prove that you are not so bad.

If you play the hero role and succeed, oddly enough the rewards do not satisfy you. Inside you will still know that the hero role is only an act, and you are much more than just that role. Although the role is not phoney, it is not the whole truth about who you are. So the success doesn't satisfy the inner part that yearned to feel fulfilled. Sometimes you may also fear being· found out as a fraud. Other people are bound to notice that you are not always the hero. Your roles fulfil an important purpose though. They have been the best you could do so far to compensate for what was unresolved in the past.

Unfortunately, some people keep repeating quite negative personal scripts again and again. Over time they begin to believe the negative traits about themselves. By thinking they are defective in some way, they create an explanation of why things never work out for them or why they deserve punishment in some form. Sometimes they hide behind these negative scripts as an excuse not to move forward in their lives.

Unhelpful Negative Scripts

An unhelpful negative script that seems to have endless variations is about not being able to attract the right partner. Having good relationships can bring so much happiness. Not having good relationships is usually due to the hidden intentions of negative scripts. Recently a middle-aged client complained to me about how she didn't have a relationship. She was always attracted to men she couldn't get. For the last eight years, none of the relationships she started felt right – there was no magic, and they didn't feel like they were going anywhere. She feared she wasn't able to sustain a relationship. Perhaps she was too boring, not attractive enough or just not interesting. To be sure, her energy was so low that despite her good looks, she was no magnet. The few men she did feel attracted to, didn't want her. Hence her negative beliefs were reinforced!

Eight years before, there had been an intense love affair – a 'Big One' – that left her with a huge heartache even though it had not lasted very long. She had been very much in love, but hadn't felt that she received love back the way she wanted it. He was distant, wouldn't communicate and seemed shut down. So she ended the relationship, even though it tore her to pieces.

However, this didn't explain where her negative script began, so she looked further back in time. She had been a tubby teenager, and her family had moved so frequently that she was always the new kid at school – making it tough to make friends. Her parents were very loving, and she adored her father, even though he was rarely home. She had always wanted his approval, but he was fairly unobtainable. The only approval he gave her was when she showed she could do things on her own. She had strong memories about how he moaned about all his dependent female relatives.

Then she mentioned that, as a teenager, she had a dream that she would never marry. Instead she would buy a farm in a very remote place in Scotland and live there all by herself. She decided that she didn't want to end up having a suburban middle class lifestyle like her parents. And of course, being so self-sufficient would certainly win her dad's approval! Her hidden intention was to prove how independent she could be to her father. Unfortunately, the results of her life indicated that her energy had obviously followed this script instead of what she consciously thought she wanted.

In time, she began to realise how these negative self-concepts of not being attractive had run in her family for several generations. Since it wasn't anyone's fault, and she had done nothing wrong, she could easily forgive herself for thinking there was something wrong with her. She was also able to let go of her old need to please her father. She then spontaneously started re-writing her script: the place in Scotland looked much sunnier, and a loving male companion joined her. They were mutually supportive – real equals! Her state became more optimistic as her future began to look so much brighter. And as her energy returned, her natural beauty began to light up from within.

The only lasting beauty is the beauty of the heart.

Rumi

The Hidden Purpose of Your Script

Just suppose for a moment that you wanted your current life script to be exactly the way it is: why might you want it that way? What hidden needs could there be? Remember this will not have been a conscious choice. Of course, if your current situation is dire, you wouldn't choose to have it that way. But what if the subconscious motive behind this script served reasons out of your awareness? Can you remember times as a child when you decided certain things about life, about yourself and about how you must live?

If you are not so sure about your script, you can get interesting insights by considering some of your favourite stories, cartoons, heroes, legends, or myths from childhood, or current favourite films and characters of today. These can give useful clues about what resonates with your deeper feelings. When you begin to appreciate what might be happening in all parts of your mind, you can begin to take full responsibility for your choices. Then you can choose to change! The following questions are designed to help reveal some possible hidden dynamics in your current script. Some of the questions may apply better than others. Stretch yourself by doing your best to find an answer to each question.

Exercise: Why have you chosen your current script to be like it is? ....

Be curious to discover possible answers for each question, and feel intuitively whether your answers make sense in some way. Sometimes you might get negative answers first. Just keep asking the questions until you discover the strange positive gains you may have been trying to get.

Positive Gain Questions
1. What are you gaining from having your script this way?
2. What are the advantages?
3. What purpose does it serve?
4. What does it give you?
5. What are you getting to be right about?
6. In what way are you indulging yourself in this situation?
7. Why have you created this?

Negative Gain Questions
1. What is it you don't have to do – as long as you run this script?
2. Who or what do you get to avoid?
3. What gift, talent or opportunity do you avoid by running this script?

4. What fear did you not have to face?
5. What dream was shattered?
6. Who or what was this an attempt to hold onto?
7. What guilt are you paying off? What did you think you did wrong?
8. In what way do you not give to your self because of this script?

Hidden Messages

1. If this script is a message to important people in your life: What could that message be and who is it for? Mother, father, partner, siblings, children, friends, colleagues, boss, professional body?
2. By having this occur, who might you be getting revenge on?
3. What does it prove – about you, about life, about men, women or something else?
4. Whose fault is it your life is like this? Who do you blame?
5. Who is it you haven't forgiven (including yourself)?
6. What might you be punishing yourself for?
7. How could your lack of self-value create this situation? If you truly believed in your self worth, how would it have been different?
8. What lesson could you be trying to learn?

If you are tempted to answer 'I don't know' or 'nothing', persist in exploring deeper. What would you answer if you did know? If you still find it difficult to answer these questions, here are some sample answers other people have discovered around particular issues:

I'm not in a good relationship because:

I'll lose my freedom, or my free time
I might have to sacrifice or compromise
I don't want to feel controlled
I want to avoid responsibility
I want to avoid boredom and sameness
I want to avoid living a stereotype
I don't trust myself to be faithful
I want to prove that (someone) hurt me

I get revenge by being alone and miserable
I want to be right about how unlovable I am
I'm terrified of intimacy and really being seen
My dream of true love was shattered
I had such terrible role models

I don't have lots of money because:
If I had lots of money, all my relatives would want handouts
I'd feel guilty about everyone who has less
I don't want to lose my friends who are not well off
I wouldn't know who my true friends are
I might become indulgent, lazy, unmotivated, shallow, greedy
I'd be classed with people I don't like
I like to think of myself as more spiritual
I want to be right about my beliefs about how money is earned
I have an excuse about not being able to do things
My dream of the world being my oyster was shattered
I don't deserve to be rich because my family was poor
I can't do better than my father

I'm not successful because:
I want to be loved for who I am, not what I do
If I was successful, I'd have to maintain that level
I'd be more afraid of having so much more to lose
It would prove that my parents did a great job if I was
I want to be right about what a failure I am
I want to avoid people finding out that I really can't do it
I am too busy proving I'm not good enough
My dream of achieving my dreams was shattered
I don't deserve it because I don't work hard enough
My family never supported me
It's a message to my father about what a bad job he did
I want to hide, not show up, stay small — safe!

I have this health issue because:
If I was healthy I'd have to show up and perform
If gives me the perfect excuse to hide behind
It means I don't have to give my gifts
Someone didn't love me enough, take care of me enough

I can hold onto whoever is taking care of me now
It proves what bad parents I had
I can indulge in feeling bad, or having a rest
I've never forgiven my mother
It helps me to avoid having intimacy
My dream of having a perfect life was shattered
I don't listen to or honour my own feelings
I deserve to be sick because I was so indulgent

I want to prove that I am – not good enough, unlovable, a failure because:
I won't have to show up, I can hide instead
If I stay small, no one can judge how well I could have done
It gives me security, an identity that is familiar
I avoid competition, effort, possible embarrassment
I want to be right about being inadequate in some way
I can blame someone else for my inadequacy
I'm indulging myself by forgetting who I really am
It means God must have made a mistake in creating me
My dream of divine love embodied in all beings was shattered
I get to avoid love, success – anything that would prove my
  worth
It proves what a bad job my parents did
I need to learn to remember who I am

Many of your answers may not sound very positive at first. Some of them might not make any sense. The mind is not always logical and reasonable. Just notice how much energy you invest in supporting these ideas. If you explore your answers further, asking the same questions, you may discover something even more surprising: most of these strange reasons are misguided attempts to attain basic needs of Love, Control, Safety and Security. See if this is true for you too.

*Misperceptions produce fear
And true perceptions foster love.*

A Course in Miracles

The Need for Love

One of our primary needs is to be loved, approved of, wanted, cared for and mothered. When this doesn't happen to children (of any age), it leads to misperceptions about lack of self worth, being unwanted, not feeling good enough, or not being included. Life then becomes a quest to prove yourself in all sorts of ways, trying to attract that attention and adoration you never received. you crave feeling accepted, approved of and cherished. You long for tenderness and intimate understanding and appreciation.

In order to fulfil this need, some people push themselves to excel, striving for the heights of success, dazzling everyone with their expertise, their beauty, their accomplishments and impressing displays of the rewards, toys, and material splendour. They believe that if they could be good enough, everyone will love them. At the opposite extreme, other people take a more revengeful route and choose to excel at being bad. Any attention is better than no attention! They choose to become cynical and hopeless about ever receiving love, so they decide to get attention in a rebellious way.

Both of these avenues of behaviour fail to satisfy or heal the underlying fear of being unworthy. The solution: re-discover your innate worthiness, innocence and lovability. Both the dazzling and dastardly behaviours are merely compensations, clever devices to hide what you really feel inside. So it is little surprise that when people lavish praise on you for all your accomplishments, or you become famous (or infamous), it doesn't reach the part that needs to be reached. Discovering the hidden dynamics requires patience and staying very open minded. If you can't imagine there might be a hidden intention behind your script, let this next story inspire you to look again.

A middle-aged woman came to see me about not being able to lose the weight she had gained after her first baby was born. She had gone from 9$^{1}/_{2}$ stone to 16 stone. No diet made any difference, despite expert advice from nutritionists and other therapists. She followed an extremely healthy diet and did regular yoga exercise, but she was now also developing thyroid and hypoglycaemic problems. Needless to say, she was extremely frustrated about not having been able to shift this weight for twenty years.

With health issues, there is usually a hidden secondary gain, some positive advantage behind the symptoms, but she was mystified when I asked her about the positive benefits of being big. At first, she could only think of the disadvantages about how much she hated being fat. She talked about how cruel and judgemental people are towards fat people. How people automatically assume that fat people are greedy and spend all their time eating junk foods. Being all too aware of the health risks, she insisted that there were no benefits at all about being big.

We discussed some of the typical secondary gains expressed through having excess weight: needing to take up more space, being important, not being overlooked, having more power, looking strong, avoiding looking too attractive, never looking weak, self protection, avoiding sex, hiding. But none of these resonated with her very strongly. She just yearned to be slim again.

Although she had a very sweet demeanour, underneath she was actually very, very angry. We traced this anger all the way back to when she was in her mother's womb. The story was that her mother didn't want to be pregnant again. Her mother was having an affair, and wanted to leave her husband. Being pregnant again made things very difficult. She wanted to get rid of this baby.

Of course, the baby in the womb could feel how unwanted she was. As extraordinary as is sounds, it seemed to her that her negative beliefs could have been formed as early as that. It made sense that she could have decided then that she was unworthy to live, how life was a struggle, how she was unimportant and therefore would have to make everything right and please everyone, that she couldn't complain, she didn't deserve to be loved or nurtured. In addition, although she didn't know what she had done wrong, it was all her fault. Obviously, there was no way she could trust this mother to nurture her, so it was unlikely she could trust any woman to nurture her (including herself).

Sure enough, after the baby was born, things went from bad to worse. Her mother did a poor job of looking after her, leaving her crying in a pram at the bottom of the garden almost every day. A few years later, her mother had another baby, and life became even more complicated. When she was twelve years old, her mother took the youngest child and walked out of the house never to return, without even saying goodbye. She was left to look after her father, do all the cooking and take care of the house.

In order to heal these intensely difficult events, she needed to find powerful reframes to see things from a more positive perspective. She found this easy until we got to the point of forgiveness. This woman had held onto so much blame and judgement against her mother, it astonished her to discover how hard it was to let go and forgive the past. The whole story of her life script had been founded on revenge for not being cared for by her mother. It was a very moving and tearful moment when she decided to let the past go. She finally found the willingness to forgive her mother.

At last her weight problem began to make some sense. Being pregnant and giving birth to her first baby must have triggered all her early memories of her own birth. Until then, these old issues had lain dormant. Ironically, she had developed her whole career around teaching mothers how to be nurturing. She showed incredible understanding and a natural gift for being a mother, probably because she had been so deprived. This was a revelation that freed her of the old anger. It may also have been that her excess weight was just a symbol of what was so important to her – a happy pregnancy. She found she could appreciate how her personal experiences in life had primed her to become the incredible specialist she is today.

> Forgiveness removes only the untrue,
> Lifting the shadows from the world and carrying it,
> Safe and sure within its gentleness.
>
> A Course in Miracles

Your ability to manifest your Dream Script into reality will depend on how honest you can be with yourself about the hidden intentions and needs behind your current life script. Until you resolve the old wounds, the patterns of your old script will continue to function and block your ability to change. The moment you let go of needing to fulfil the hidden intentions behind your current life script, you can begin creating miracles in your life. You may be wondering how you would know if you had already healed and resolved the old wounds. Just ask yourself if there is anyone you feel anything but love for? Notice if there are any reservations, withholding, or denials. Check out any past situation where you still feel judgement or blame. When you can see every person as innocent (including yourself), you have resolved the past issue.

Seeing People as Innocent

There may be some incident that you feel justified in being angry about. When someone has made a terrible mistake, behaved badly, and hurt others, it can be very hard to forgive. But if you can imagine stepping into their shoes for a moment, and feel what it must have been like to live their life, this different perspective can help you to understand. Imagine them being an innocent baby, growing up with the parents, schools and experiences they had. Think about the influences that have made them the way they are. How could they possibly think or behave any differently? In their model of the world, everything they did made sense and served some purpose. They, too, will be running unhelpful scripts with hidden intentions that command them to act in certain ways. Once you grasp the truth of what it might have been like to be that person in the problem situation, you can begin to find grounds for forgiveness.

It is also very helpful to separate the person from their behaviours, beliefs and actions. If you can imagine that inside each person is the tiny little child they once were, it is easier to realise that back then they were totally innocent. Whatever they learned, however they were treated, and how they grew up to be, might have been full of mistakes. Their current behaviour is just the sum total of not learning from those mistakes. Bad behaviour is never acceptable, but it is always possible to forgive the person behind it.

A principle that helps this understanding is: 'People always make the best choices available to them, given their map of the world.' What this means is that people are always doing their best, even though that 'best' might not be good enough in your books. In their world, they are limited by what knowledge, skills and understanding they have. Although you may think they could have done better, in fact, what they gave was their best. Of course, this also applies to you. Can you ever do better than your best? Haven't you always done the best you could, despite making mistakes? In fact, isn't it true that you usually only knew you were making a mistake AFTER the event? Do your best now at discovering where you might have a hidden need for forgiveness. This is not about condoning bad behaviour, it is about learning the lesson, forgiving and moving on.

Exercise: Healing the need for approval................................

1. Are there any areas in your life where you are always trying to get approval, love, admiration, respect, understanding, appreciation? Identify all the different ways you do that. Recognise even the smallest places where the need for love and approval triggers various behaviours to try to get it. There is nothing wrong with wanting love and approval in any form.
2. You might notice that there is a particular type of love and approval you think you don't get enough of. Trace this back in time, and collect all the various different instances where you felt this lack.
3. Find the earliest example, the first incident that could have created the belief and pattern of behaviour. Notice what was going on then. Notice who else was involved.
4. Notice any judgments that could have been made. Notice what you decided about the other person(s), yourself, about men, women, what you could expect of life, success, what you deserved, about God.
5. Step into the shoes of each person one at a time, and imagine what life must have been like for them. Imagine what sort of upbringing they had, what sort of knowledge and wisdom was available to them. Imagine how they were feeling at the time. Imagine what possible behaviours they were actually capable of at that time.
6. Remember that: 'People always make the best choice available according to their map of the world'. Remove any ideas about how they could have done it differently or better. What they did was their best choice at that time. This also applies to you.

7. Is it possible for you to forgive them now? Could you let go of the judgement, blame and anger around this early event?
8. Access your Heart: What else could you learn that might help you to let go of this early need for love and approval? What would happen if you applied these lessons to all the other incidents in your life that have a similar flavour?

Reframing

Have you ever noticed that almost everyone thinks they act with good intentions? Sometimes the intention is only for their own benefit or protection, but frequently these actions are justified as being the best for others too. Occasionally people will admit that they acted in anger, or with greed, and possibly feel guilty enough to apologise or have regrets. But few people accurately assess whether their heart or their ego lies behind most of their actions.

Remember that 'Behind every behaviour is a positive intention'. What is important to realise is that, when a person behaves badly, they may still be behaving with a positive intention in their limited understanding, or corrupted model of the world. They are innocently choosing to do what feels right for them. They don't know better, or have never been taught to think differently, or they simply do not have the necessary awareness or skills.

When you understand where people are coming from, it can help a lot towards being able to communicate better and work together. In order to fully forgive someone for bad behaviour, it can be crucial to appreciate when, where and why a person chose to be like that. The vital tool of 'Reframing' can help you think from a more healing perspective. Reframing changes the viewpoint, meaning or context of a certain behaviour or idea. Instead of getting caught up with what is being said on the surface, it can be extremely useful to tune into the underlying needs. The following simple questions can help you get a better idea of the positive intentions behind anyone's behaviour.

Exercise: How to 'Reframe' and get more useful perspectives ....

Practice asking and answering the following reframe questions about an incident where you still feel upset:

1 What positive intention could this idea or behaviour have?
2. How is it possible they could believe that or behave that way (what overall belief must they have that supports that?
3. Where in the world could this idea or behaviour be useful? With whom?
4. When could this idea or behaviour be useful? (past, present, future)
5. What part of this idea or behaviour could be good here and now?
6. What will happen to them if they continue to think this way?
7. Why did they think or do this – for what purpose?
8. What would happen if they thought or did the opposite?

Example:

Behaviour: Someone is being abusive, attacking and angry.

1. **Positive intentions:** they want to get their way, be right, have power, control, domination, get their needs met, hide their inadequacy.
2. **Overall belief:** since they never got what they wanted, or never felt respected, they have to fight for it, only violence works, the mightiest always win.
3. **Where useful:** possibly in a real battle situation; when standing up for what is true or what needs defending.
4. **When useful:** it might have worked as a baby to get more attention or care, it might work now in situations where threats are effective, there may be times in the future where anger needs to be expressed.
5. **What part useful:** being in touch with one's feelings and recognising anger as a signal that one's values or boundaries are not respected.
6. **Consequence:** increased blood pressure, other health issues; poor relationships and lack of rapport.
7. **Purpose:** get respect, attention, protect their space or position, win.
8. **Opposite behaviour:** in their map of the world, if they didn't use anger and abuse: they would be walked all over; be weak; lose respect, power, authority; and not get their needs met.

Being Objective

A common assumption that confuses many people is that they occupy an objective middle ground of thinking. Many people believe that the truth is somehow separate, provable, measurable, and justified by evidence and reasoned argument. They forget that these 'truths' usually support only one map of the world – usually their own map! Since no one is all-seeing, all-knowing, it is safe to assume that these truths are usually based on limited sensory input. But it is amazing how the ideas, values, and beliefs that develop as a consequence are held as sacrosanct. People become so convinced and attached to these truths that they will defend them unto death.

Perhaps you've found yourself in arguments with people who hold an opposing view to your own and wondered how they could maintain they were right in the face of overwhelming evidence to the contrary? Or maybe you have watched the TV news in different countries and discovered how each country reports its version of 'truth'. On a world scale it is unfortunate and very worrying how often this phenomenon occurs. Politics and the media selectively choose evidence to justify some action or point of view. As people argue the pros and cons of some action or inaction, few people search for the deeper level of truth, justice or humanity.

As well as ferreting out the positive hidden intention, sometimes you will need to access a deeper level of truth. If you want to unblock what holds you back from manifesting your Dream Script into reality, it might be necessary to look beyond what you normally hold to be right, and get in touch with what is really true for you. Here is a story that illustrates what this means.

An irate husband, who had been made redundant at work, came in complaining bitterly about all of his wife's short comings. Their house was always untidy, she bullied him and the children, she was irresponsible about paying the bills, and spent money on extravagances. He related story after story of unreasonable behaviour, fights, and how intolerable his life had become. His anger was all about how she needed to change, because she was the cause of all his bad feelings. As he continued to feed his anger by blaming his wife for his bad feelings, it grew to the point of wanting to give up and get a divorce. He didn't realise how focusing on his wife provided a neat distraction to divert attention away from his low self-esteem and his issue about creating a new career.

Although he was convinced by the reasoning and evidence of each complaint, it was also obvious that he dearly loved his wife and children more than anything in the world. So I asked him why he was focusing on complaints instead of remembering his true feelings? What he really wanted by being so angry, was to be listened to, to be loved, and to be accepted despite his work predicament. His deeper needs actually had little to do with the family, and much more to do with old childhood wounds.

He was willing to explore an old misunderstanding from three years old, a time when he felt unwanted and rejected by his father. He had decided then that 'life was hard work', and that he would have to prove his worth in order to get his father's love. Since that time he had spent his whole life struggling to make it in a career he didn't even like, in order to impress his father. After accessing his own inner, deeper truth, he realised his real worth, how loved he was by everyone and how it didn't matter whether or not people gave him attention. From this perspective, he was able to reconnect with the love for his wife and children and all the negative complaints evaporated.

Every minute you are angry, you lose sixty seconds of happiness.

Ralph Waldo Emerson

Handling Anger

Sometimes it is easy to feel justified in being angry. Maybe someone has behaved badly, overstepped the mark, violated your values, or trespassed on your territory. It may just be a 'bad day': one of those times when everything seems to go wrong. Your buttons get pushed and before you think, you react in anger.

For some people, every day seems to be a 'bad day'. They get labelled short tempered because they develop this behaviour as a habit. They seem to walk around in a constant state of anger, just looking for something to attack. Road rage is a good example. But more subtle forms are less easy to identify. Anger includes cynical remarks, complaining, criticising, nagging, being sarcastic, and being unco-operative on purpose. Sometimes anger can be expressed just with a look or a sneer. Showing up late or not showing up at all can also be an expression of anger. Constantly doubting that things could work out well, often adds more energy to the negative qualities and becomes 'bad attitude'. It seems to serve no good purpose.

Anger destroys good feeling and creates bad atmospheres. Outbursts and attacks are not easily forgotten. The more violent the attack, the more other people get scared and feel they need to protect themselves. No matter how well you make up afterwards, a scar is formed. Trust is lost and fear reigns. The irony is that the hidden cause behind anger is also fear. You feel angry when what is important to you is not respected. Someone has trampled on your values, or trespassed on your boundaries. You fear that you have already been attacked, so anger seems like the best way to defend and protect you.

The truth is, anger can be one of your most useful allies. Have you ever noticed that your feelings of anger can surface quicker than your mind can identify what you are angry about? If you notice the first signs of anger: feeling hot, grinding your teeth, breathing faster, tight neck muscles, blood starting to pump, you can recognise any one of these as a warning signal. Ask yourself immediately, 'What important value do I think has just been violated?' Then check out whether that is based on fact or not. You might have misjudged the situation. If you can identify exactly how or where you are feeling under attack, then it might be possible to design better ways to protect yourself more appropriately. Here's a story about handling anger.

An attractive artist confessed that she often felt very upset. Her core problem was that she was not good at receiving criticism or being 'told' what to do. In fact, she easily became enraged! It sounded like whatever she said or did was not enough. Feeling defensive, protective and cagey, she would reply (with bad attitude) 'I'm TRYING!' These situations caused uncomfortable feelings in her chest and left her with a sense that she was never good enough. She often thought she couldn't win no matter what she did, and then she felt helpless and frustrated.

This bad attitude had been with her for a long time. As far back as she could remember, whatever she did never seemed enough. Whatever she had said at school had never been right. Her family were all strong-willed people who loved her, but she was never acknowledged for doing well. Although she rarely raised her voice, her intonation clearly indicated she carried a lot of anger around with her.

Remembering that, 'You are never upset for the reason you think you are', we started wondering just where these bad feelings had originally come from. It was obvious that the current situation was more a trigger than a cause. Her reactions were clearly out of proportion to what was happening. Even she had to admit that she was verging on becoming a rage-aholic inside, even if she didn't openly express her anger outside. She had become adept at expressing her anger in passive aggressive ways: a look, a tone of voice, withdrawing her energy into a stony silence, or making prickly comments.

Underneath the anger was a lot of old pain, plus the feeling of being helpless, hopeless and worthless. The old pain was so deep, it seemed to go back through several generations on both sides of her family. She intuitively daydreamed an image of her great, great grandmother sitting at a table in a black dress with her hair pulled back in a bun. This woman was not allowed to go out, or to do anything much. Although she was not unwell, she was such a non-conformist that perhaps people thought she was crazy. Her child had been taken away from her because somehow her behaviour was not acceptable, not normal. Perhaps she was too intense, energetic and happy – her wildness frightened people. Maybe they thought she was a witch.

She wondered what positive beliefs or lessons might have helped the miserable woman in this situation. Her Heart responded by affirming that this woman was not only OK, and had a good heart, but that she was an important part of the universe. She was created to be just the way she was, and was not to be judged as right or wrong. She was definitely good enough. The people who judged her probably acted out of jealousy or fear, but she could remember that she was loved. Her Heart reminded her to pay attention to her own needs rather than to the demands of others. All these ideas helped both her and her great, great grandmother feel more calm and comfortable.

After collecting all these useful ideas, she thought of several other relatives who needed similar help. She felt happy to share her new wisdom, beginning to believe for herself how essential it was to be who she was. When she fully re-connected with her true self, feeling her worth, knowing she was an important part of the universe, all of her self judgement melted away and there was no longer any desire to be angry.

Deep within you is everything that is perfect, ready to radiate through you and out into the world.

A Course in Miracles

What is your most typical way of expressing anger? Are you a person who shouts and expresses anger in a very outward way? Or are you a person who never expresses anger openly, but uses passive aggressive ways to let people know how you feel? Or are you someone who believes you never get angry? Some people claim that they don't 'do' anger at all. Usually that means that they don't express it openly, or with a raised voice. Remember that anger can be expressed by your actions, your gestures, your eyes and certain voice tones. Cynicism, sarcasm, withdrawal, non-communication and being absent are quite powerful expressions of anger.

Remember that your genuine feelings of anger are valuable and worthy of your attention. Your anger, like all your feelings, has a purpose and needs to be heard. Learn to listen to your anger, find out what the signal is trying to alert you to. Your anger can be your best friend, letting you know in a flash that something about a situation stinks. If you learn to use your anger wisely and work with it compassionately, it can be a precious tool. Your feelings react faster than your mind can analyse any situation.

If you think you rarely get angry, here is a list of other forms of anger that might be easier to recognise: being cross, irritated, frustrated, impatient, exasperated, indignant, annoyed, furious, hostile, disgruntled, mean, vicious, withdrawn, cold, cutting, sarcastic, cynical, depressed, revengeful, as well as feeling animosity, hatred, rage, wrath and violence.

Exercise: Dealing with anger ....

Do you suspect you carry around a lot of anger? How often do you have patches where you find yourself taking it out on other people? Here are some tips:

1. First acknowledge that you are feeling angry, and get curious to know and understand what the real cause is. Chances are, there are good reasons for you to have felt like this. Honour that.

2. Notice the language you use when you are amplifying a situation: words like 'Never, Always, Everyone, All, Every time, Forever. Notice how these presuppose that what is happening now can never change – question that by remembering that no one can predict the future. It can't possibly be true Always and Forever.

3. Detect whether you or someone else is making rules. You should/shouldn't do this. You have to do that. You ought to, must, can't do that. Look for the exceptions to these rules. Maybe they don't apply in all situations. Where are these rules NOT true?

4. Are there judgements involved? There may be both explicit and implicit value judgements. What are they? Who is making that observation? What are the exceptions? Is it a question of right or wrong, good or bad? Life is seldom so simple.

5. If this angry feeling is a bit of a habit, when did it start? Anger has the positive purpose of protecting and defending what is valuable and important. What or who was being protected back then? If a situation comes to mind, clarify the story and ask your Heart for the positive lessons that would have helped. Let the anger go.

6. Reaffirm the truth of your worth. Choose to connect with your Heart. Let any judgements melt away and enjoy the peace that brings.

If you have followed all the exercises so far, you should have gained some new perspectives and deeper understanding about what is going on in your life right now, and about what used to hold you back. Maybe some of the blocks to your success have already lifted. As you learn how to recognise and deal with guilt and anger, you may also start to feel more innocent and at peace. These are qualities that begin to attract good things happening in your life. Imagine being able to attract all the elements of your Dream Script just like a magnet. But if you have uncovered some issues that do not yet feel resolved, move on to the next chapter and discover how to transform difficult events.

Chapter Summary:

Principles:

Every behaviour is useful in some context.
People always make the best choices available to them at the time.

Checklist:

1. Just suppose you wanted your current script to be the way it is, why?
2. What are the:
   a. Positive Gains?
   b. Negative Gains?
   c. Messages?
3. Take yourself through the steps to feeling more Love, Acceptance and Appreciation.
4. Use the 'Reframing' questions to elicit different perspectives for deeper and more healing understandings.
5. Understand, honour and let go of any kind of excess anger you might have.

6

Healing the Source

It is enough to heal the past
And make the future free.
It is enough to let the present
Be accepted as it is.

A COURSE IN MIRACLES

If the human mind is like a magnificent computer, there must be crossed wires, or a software problem somewhere. Or maybe there are brain computer viruses that interfere with its ability to function properly. How else can you explain why people will go out of their way to avoid, prevent, or hide from the very things they want the most? So often, people know exactly what they want, and they appear to do everything they can to achieve that happening, only to sabotage their own efforts. When they receive nothing but frustration and disappointment in return, it is heartbreaking. If people fail enough times, they often give up, and lose heart. They don't know what stops them. They don't know how to find a way through.

You may think you know exactly what stops you. A challenging work opportunity may trigger fears of being found lacking. A chance to show up and shine, raises the risk of being exposed as a fraud. A possibility to perform and be creative, suddenly breeds stage fright. Even more personal situations, like actually choosing to love someone, can cause terror, hiding and shrinking away. Fear, in some disguise, seems directly linked to a specific cause you can identify. But you are never upset for the reason you think you are. Often those fears are out of proportion to the situation. Although the trigger for a particular fear may be obvious, the underlying cause may be hidden. Learning

Compassionate Coaching techniques can help discover the real causes and heal them.

Exploring the Edges of Your Comfort Zone

Are you aware of the limits of your own comfort zone? Have you ever been tempted to stay with what is familiar and predictable – the comfort of the devil you know so well? Have you ever felt terrified of being found deficient in some way? Do you procrastinate about the projects that once inspired you at the start, but now, somehow, you just can't complete? Maybe there was a time when you refused to stand up and share who you came to be. Perhaps you are someone who always prefers to avoid confrontation. And who do you know who runs away from honest sharing and true intimacy? In the past it may have felt so much easier to stay small and just dream of what could have been achieved. It may have seemed the best way to avoid the possible embarrassment and pain of failure. Are you ready now to learn how to heal these fears?

If you blame some external factor for holding you back, especially if you feel powerless to change it, then you'll feel helpless. The more responsibility you can take for your life, the more you will regain the power to create what you want. When you no longer blame something outside yourself as a reason for things not happening, you are forced to look inside. You can learn how to make inner changes that really make a difference.

A trap to avoid, however, is thinking there is an internal saboteur holding you back. If you are consciously doing everything you can to achieve your dreams, and nothing works, it can be tempting to think there is an internal alien preventing your success. However, even if that were the case, it would still be a part of YOU. No matter how horrible or destructive it might sound, welcome it into your understanding, find out what it wants, and why it wants to hold you back. What you resist, persists. What you fight against and try to suppress, grows bigger and more rebellious. When you understand the deeper issues, it is much easier to find a healing path. If you can respect and honour the intentions of any awkward feelings, they can just exist, without having to control your behaviour.

Oddly enough, all your fears of being small, deficient, lacking or a fraud may be just a cover-up. There could be something even more terrifying than failure. While you focus on the fears that hold you back from achieving your dreams, you spend all your attention and energy dealing with what turns out to be nothing more than negative illusions. After you gain the wisdom and discover the positive intentions that heal the old stories, these fears evaporate. However, be prepared, because there could be deeper fears underneath waiting to surface!

Fear of Success

The truth is that most people are more afraid of success than of failure. If they were to achieve the life of their dreams, then they would have so much more to lose! Would they be able to maintain their new level of expertise? Success starts to sound like never-ending effort, obligation, demands, and hard work. Once obtained, it would be so much more embarrassing and humiliating to lose it than never to have had it in the first place. So many people choose to keep themselves small, and never take the risk.

If they reached success, would friends and relatives get jealous? It might upset the very relationships that supported them and made it possible. How would it be possible to handle other people's reactions? Would people still love them for who they are, or only for their abundance and success? Would it become hard to know who was a true friend? Some people fear that success means they would always be looking over their shoulder waiting for attack, waiting for people to steal from them or cheat them. Could they trust anyone anymore?

What if they really had the good health, fantastic fitness or the perfect body, what would they have to do then! What bigger demands, what challenges would they have to face? If other people found them more attractive, would they be able to handle that with integrity? Do they trust themselves?

What more would they expect of themselves once they reached the first rung of success? Would they just set higher goals and keep striving even harder? Or would they lose all their motivation because there was nothing left to aim for anymore? Even worse, do they *deserve* to have the life of their dreams? Could they really be powerful and not get big headed or corrupted?

> *Our deepest fear is not that we are inadequate. Our deepest fear is that we are powerful beyond measure. It is our light, not our darkness, that most frightens us. We ask ourselves, who am I to be brilliant, gorgeous, talented and fabulous? Actually, who are you not to be?*
>
> Marianne Williamson

The previous chapters have explored the hidden underlying needs, the positive intentions, and the possible gains that keep people locked into dysfunctional scripts. In order to make way for your Dream Script, it may be necessary to re-visit and heal whatever type of fear emerges from examining your current script. Please remember to stay connected with your Heart, your giftedness and your purpose, in order to stay in balance.

Underlying Dynamics

Remember whatever is happening in your current script that is not of your conscious choosing, must be coming from your unconscious mind. This is the part of your mind that creates your dreams at night. It also constructs bizarre reasons and justifications for all the decisions you ever made going back to childhood. The unconscious mind incorporates ideas and concepts from films, books, magazines, or newspapers. It isn't interested whether or not you believe in these ideas, because it uses them as metaphors for other meanings anyway. Therefore the underlying dynamics of your story may include limiting beliefs, bad decisions, vows, negative emotions, even curses that go back in time through your family tree. Unhelpful attitudes combine several of these qualities, and can be handed down from generation to generation. Your children may be learning lessons like these from you right now. If a story goes back in time, the original source needs to be explored. Often it is useful to think of this metaphorically. Because your memory of the past may or may not be accurate, it's best to think: it's just a story. In fact, even if you believe the story to be true, remember you have only one version of it. Treat it as 'just a story'.

Even if you were to choose a childhood fairytale or an ancient Greek myth, whatever story you resonate with will reveal hidden structures of how your unconscious mind thinks. Remember your unconscious mind loves the realm of symbols and metaphors. Just think of the incredible stories it makes up in your dreams at night. Facts, characters and details disguise important clues in dreams. But what is revealed in the plot, no matter how exaggerated or bizarre, contains similar themes and feelings to what needs to be unravelled, unpicked and undone in your own unconscious mind.

> *What you think you are is a belief to be undone.*
>
> A Course in Miracles

Traumatic emotional events during childhood are often the source of limiting beliefs, ideas and decisions. However, some unhelpful attitudes can be inherited, passed down from generation to generation. Children tend to copy their parents' demeanour, expressions, gestures and how they express themselves. Unconsciously, they also pick up the ideas, values and beliefs that go with them. Please remember the object of this exercise is not about looking to put blame somewhere else. By exploring an earlier cause, you can gain new perspectives of understanding, and appreciate why people behaved the way they did. Parents usually do the best they can to teach their children how to fit into society. Whatever their experience, whatever their beliefs – these become their idea of the norm. In an effort to foster good manners and behaviour, parents instil 'rules' based on their model of the world. Often, different forms of punishment are used as deterrents for breaking these rules. Unfortunately, punishments can get out of hand, ranging from a withdrawal of all love and attention, to full-blown, violent physical attack.

Children learn more from example than they do from what parents say. They learn from modelling their parents' behaviour and can be oblivious to any positive intentions of their parents. A young child does not have the capacity to understand why the parent is behaving violently all of a sudden. It can be frightening and confusing. The parent's love then seems unpredictable and the child begins to feel very insecure. In an effort to restore the good feelings again, the child tries to be compliant: to be a good boy or a good girl. If that doesn't work, however, the child might decide that bad attention is better than no attention and sets out to be a bad boy or bad girl. It's surprising how much a normal, uneventful 'happy childhood' can create unhelpful patterns of thinking and beliefs that persist to adulthood.

A good example of how the real cause of stuck patterns of behaviour can originate in childhood, is this story told by a very experienced facilitator and trainer. Despite teaching Positive Outcomes himself, he felt he needed help exploring some of the hidden dimensions behind his health issue. He had been HIV positive for over eight years. 'Isn't it funny,' he said, 'that the positive state is actually the negative!' Of course, he had done masses of personal development work to uncover what his illness meant to him. In his case, being HIV positive was a 'Wake Up Call' for him to change his direction and life style. It became a catalyst for working on himself and dealing with his guilt. Although he had benefited from all the work he had done, he had recently lost two stone very suddenly. He secretly worried that this might be the first side effect of the HIV. Most of the time he believed he had such a strong constitution that he could not only put the weight back on, but also heal completely.

His guilt started when he was a teenager, worrying about what people would think of him for being gay. He wasn't comfortable about being gay. He could never tell his father! After his father died, he finally told his mother and sister, but their carefully measured affirmative reactions didn't feel honest to him.

Living with his mother for forty-seven years, he described her as always reliable, always there, and very safe to be with. However, she could also be very opinionated and procedural. There was never much love demonstrated. What he got was a sense that he 'must be a good boy' in order to deserve love. Of course, no matter what he did, he still received very little love. Suddenly, as he described this, an extraordinary amount of anger welled up inside him! He had been SUCH a good boy – he scored himself 9 out of 10. Yet he always had to walk on eggshells around his mother. He had to stay constantly alert, since whatever he did, could be wrong. He couldn't be enthusiastic or too happy – her number one rule was 'don't show any emotions!'

His anger seemed to be stored just behind his belly button. He wondered if this could be a link with his illness. The anger was certainly stimulating lots of adrenalin being released. But the idea that he 'must be a good boy' had become such an identity, he didn't want to let it go. It felt safe, familiar – the status quo of his comfort zone. Without this belief running his life, how would he know what was right? He might get things wrong! He wanted to avoid any unknown territory. He didn't want to be out of control. Being flexible felt frightening!

Because his anger seemed a bit out of proportion to his childhood memories we delved deeper to discover whether there was another cause. He was the second child of his parents. His sister was fourteen years older. When his mother had discovered she was two months pregnant with him, she was not happy. She didn't really want another child and didn't cope well with the idea. But her belief was that, 'She had to do the right thing and give birth.' She was very angry to be pregnant at her advanced age. And she felt extremely guilty! Everyone would know that she had had sex – what would people think! She worried about not having enough money, and what life would be like with another baby to look after. Of course, all of these ideas and feelings flooded into the tiny baby inside her. There are no secrets between a mother and a baby in the womb.

Beginning to realise how he might have swallowed some of his mother's anger and guilt, he was now able to make more sense of his own feelings. He added his Heart's understanding to heal the little baby part of his unconscious memory. He installed beliefs he felt were true for him: Love is not dependent on anything. It's OK to feel and express emotions appropriately. Honesty is wonderful. Never get yourself into a situation where money is a problem. It's OK to make mistakes and learn from them. Remember to trust, and that whatever happens is meant to happen.

While his inner changes continued to integrate into a new, more peaceful persona, he began unravelling the layers of trying so hard to be a 'good boy' and win his mother's love. With less anger stimulating his fight or flight adrenal response, he felt that his immune system might have more energy to work on healing his illness. It felt like an important step forward.

Every situation, properly perceived, becomes an opportunity to heal.

A Course in Miracles

Identifying the original source of unhelpful ideas, beliefs, feelings and attitudes may not make sense at first. Don't expect to remember a cause, or for everything to seem logical. The unconscious mind thinks laterally and metaphorically. Its favourite realms are legend, fantasy, myth, fairies, demons and dragons. If you trust whatever springs into your mind as a story, just be curious about how that story is structured. What is important about the theme or the plot? What are the underlying needs, and what lesson most needs to be learned? In some way, how does this story reflect what is going on in your life right now?

Another example of being stuck in old patterns is the story of a very successful businessman I worked with who was running a classic action-packed race track movie script. He believed life was so precious that he had to go as fast as he could to fit as much as possible into every minute. He spoke so quickly that many people could not keep up with his words or ideas. As his brain sped along at the rate of knots, he had to keep going faster and faster just to keep up with his mind. Although he enjoyed the speed, there were a few things missing from his script. He found it difficult to access his memory or use the more creative side of his brain. Even he noticed that his communication left many people in the dust! Not surprisingly there was no leading lady in his movie. Rather like 007, many ladies appeared, but none of them could keep up with his pace for very long.

What he actually wanted – since he had everything else – was to have a wonderful relationship with a partner he could trust totally and feel free to have fun and laugh with. What became obvious when listening to him talk, was that a lot of his conversation sounded like a ping pong match. He loved nothing better than a lively discussion. He would play devil's advocate just for the sport of making a debate. It made him feel like something was happening rather than being bored. He didn't care too much about winning, so he would continue mismatching in an analytical way just for fun. He admitted that he used to be a verbal bully, but he stopped that when he realised it didn't win him friends.

This habit of mismatching and creating analytical debates had been with him for a long time. We traced it back to a series of incidents when he was a small boy. Back then, his father had been the authoritarian bully who struggled to keep his two older sisters in line. One of his older sisters was a real rebel and the fights between her and her father often became rather ugly, and sometimes violent. Watching this at only seven years old, he discovered that if he distracted his father with an interesting argument, it took the heat off his sister. Consequently, he perfected this talent whenever the situation called for it. Later at boarding school it also came in handy. As this imprint was reinforced many times, it became part of his unconscious behaviour pattern.

Luckily, he was aware of the effects it was having on other people, and he genuinely wanted to change his script. Together, we explored his past, locating an early childhood event where he first began to think about running so fast. He was willing to review this particular event and explore each person in the family and their perspective about what happened. Some of his major realisations were about understanding that his father hadn't known how to react any differently, and may have felt very alone and unsupported in his role in the family. He imagined giving a gift to his father as a metaphor of what was needed: an hourglass to symbolise slowing down and taking it easy! What the whole family had in common was a need for patience, and a sense of being wanted and worthwhile. As he experienced each perspective fully, and received the gifts and understandings for himself, the shift in him was obvious. He relaxed and even began to speak at a more normal pace. It was then more possible for him to have different gears: to be able to think, act and speak quickly whenever it was necessary, and also to have a low gear for better conversations and more intimacy.

Things do not change, we change.

Henry David Thoreau

If there is an event in your past that needs a healing perspective, use the following exercise. You can use it for as many issues as you need to heal.

Exercise: Healing past issues ....

1. First identify the negative feelings, or limiting beliefs that you have in your current life script. Use the feelings to guide your unconscious mind back to other similar events, not stopping too long at remembered situations, until you get back to the original cause. Ideally, your original cause will be a time BEFORE you can remember, usually before the age of seven. Then it will be much easier to view it as just a story. If you don't know what the original cause was, just let your unconscious mind make up a story!

2. Write down the story of whatever you imagine and whoever was involved from a cool observer point of view. It might help to set out a chair for each of the people involved or you could put pairs of shoes on the floor to represent the position of each different person.

3. Stepping back from the situation, observe it objectively and appreciate how this event helped you to develop certain beliefs, qualities and ways of behaviour that have made you the way you are today, for better or worse. Notice that the negative effects an experience may have generated, have often led to the development of certain strengths. Remember there is always the opportunity for further learning and enlightenment.

4. Step into the shoes of one of the other people involved in the event. Note what made this person behave the way they did, and why they thought or believed that way. If you don't know, just imagine what their whole life must have been like to cause them to behave like this. How were they feeling? What were their positive intentions?

5. Re-evaluate the event from the observer position again, and notice any changes in how you feel. If possible, with your new insights and understanding, forgive the person for any

behaviour that was unhelpful. Use your ability to reframe, and intuit what hidden gains and needs they had. What qualities or understandings did they need? When you can identify those qualities, could you imagine giving them to that person? Present them as a metaphorical 'gift'.

6. Step back into the shoes of that other person and let them receive the gift. Notice how differently they now behave in the situation.

7. Repeat steps 3–5 with every other person (including yourself) involved in the event, even if they were not physically present. Sometimes, someone's absence means as much as someone's actions.

8. Re-visit the event by stepping into your own shoes one last time, but now with all the new understandings and forgiveness. How differently do you feel? How could you behave or react in that situation now? How could you re-write the script for this story now?

9. Celebrate your new sense of appreciation for the understandings and the positive roles that everyone played in assisting your development. Staying connected with all these new lessons, re-assess the situations throughout your life that had similar dynamics, and notice how they begin to feel easier. Imagine how differently you will be able to handle events like this in the future.

....

Unreachable Goals

Your current script might reveal some quality that feels out of reach or unobtainable. Does any of it seem impossible? Maybe you would just like to have more of a particular attribute. What is it you want to do that eludes you? Notice how you feel about that, or what emotions are connected with it. Has anyone else in your family history had this problem? Where might this idea have originated? If you did achieve this or reach this height, would you be disloyal to anyone? Sometimes there is an unspoken rule in families that everyone should know their place and not step beyond their station. Even after parents are long gone, some people are still maintaining loyalty to their memories by holding themselves back, staying small, or not succeeding in some way.

No one can make you feel inferior without your consent.
Eleanor Roosevelt

You can only feel disappointed with some aspect of your life if you are making a comparison to some ideal. You can only feel unhappy if you want things to be different from how they are. Your current script may not be bringing you happiness. If you know what you are not happy about, what would make you happy? This important information can assist you in creating a better script. Once you have discovered your old concepts of what would make you happy, you can re-assess your situation. Is this really what you want? Does this really inspire you? Would you be achieving this to delight yourself, or to please others? Are you trying to prove something? Consider the possibility that if certain things haven't happened, it is because on some level, you didn't want them to happen anyway.

For example, a striking looking young film producer said her particular block was the 'men thing'. Like many people, she felt confused about the balance between men and women in relationships. Expectations about levels of satisfaction have changed, and because both sexes have more freedom and choice than ever before, no one is willing to compromise. Advertising and the media have intensified romantic ideals, causing many people to fall into competitive thinking and behaviour, chasing perfect looks, super slim bodies, youth, success and chemistry. When these ideals are not met, people either reject the people they judge negatively, or judge themselves as inadequate.

It had been six years since this particular woman had dated anyone, despite reading many self help books and working through her own personal issues. She noticed that her pattern was to fall in love with men who were emotionally unavailable. Then she would try to get them to love her. 'It was like drug addiction,' she said. 'I'd project onto them all kinds of attractiveness, intelligence, and believe that they were really "there for me". But the reality was that they didn't appreciate me at all, often put me down and didn't even respect my feelings.' Ironically the men she was attracted to were often chasing other women who were not interested in them!

In the past, her relationships ended with a great deal of anger, what she described as 'torch and burn' behaviour! More recently she had become much more at peace, but she still felt like there was a monster growling over her head, silently screaming and distracting her from her work.

For years she believed she was unattractive and overweight. She felt she just couldn't do the 'feminine thing'. She could never wear a tight t-shirt! She didn't want that kind of attention. She wanted to be liked and loved for her brain, not her body, and she felt embarrassed at the thought of exposing herself. Although she had beautiful skin, she was terribly self-conscious about the thousands of moles she had. She feared that if she tried to be feminine, men would 'smell a rat'! It felt like she was playing at something that was way above her head.

As an only child, she had never received any feedback or encouragement about being attractive. Everyone in her family was thin, and her father equated 'thin with rich' and 'fat with peasant'. Because she was not thin, they encouraged her to be smart and sporty. Any attempts she made to wear lipstick or mini skirts were met with criticism: 'You look like a prostitute!' Just talking about these issues was enough to bring up waves of self-attack and anger towards her parents, towards men and even towards God.

She said this anger felt like an octopus stuck in her throat. We traced the origin of it back three generations, but it could have been many more. Her great grandmother had felt totally trapped by her circumstances, living in a tiny two-up, two-down house, looking after the children and keeping up the pretences of 'good people'. Her incredible frustration stemmed from a total lack of emotion, passion, and satisfaction in her relationship. She felt trapped with no way out.

Re-writing the script for her great grandmother, the young film producer was able to fathom many inner truths to reframe the difficult situation. Her Heart's advice focused on loving her kids, loving everyone, loving the seasons and loving life itself. If she could have spoken to that great grandmother, she would have encouraged her to express her passion without fear of being ashamed. She could start small, with a smile. Letting others into her life would help her to have a better perspective and emerge from her 'shell'. It was amazing to hear her talk about the importance of accepting herself, feeling and honouring her own feelings and being a vehicle for love.

As she considered the lives of her great grandmother, grandmother and mother, she realised she had absorbed some of her mother's deep sadness and loneliness – that sense of being alone in a world where no one understands you. The sense of abandonment and loss weighed heavily down the left side of her body. Big tears flowed as she resonated with the sense of self-pity and melancholy. But once again, she asked her Heart for deeper understandings about getting in touch with her creativity, knowing she is here for a purpose, which will become clear to her in time. She appreciated that this lonely experience would teach her sensitivity and awareness. Her love and support for her mother felt overwhelming, and it more than made up for those over-protective criticisms she may have received as a child. Perhaps she could now begin to give herself permission to be the beautiful woman she always deserved to be.

We are not searching for the meaning of life, we are searching for the experience of being alive.

Joseph Campbell

Notice that it is important to continue to use all the skills from previous chapters to find ways to reframe and heal the original source of the beliefs, ideas and feelings that hold you back in your current script, especially accessing your Heart for guidance. Here is a list of the principles covered so far:

....

Begin with a positive outcome.
The meaning of the communication is the response you get.
Think big and stay flexible about your ideas for happiness.
The person who is most flexible is most likely to get their desired results.
Let go of wanting too much.
Let go of attachment to having it be a certain way.
You already have all the gifts and resources you need to succeed.
Be kind to yourself.
Avoid the traps of overwhelm and perfectionism.

Behind every behaviour and choice is a positive intention.
You choose who directs your script.
You can re-connect with your innocence.
Every behaviour is, or was, useful in some context.
People always make the best choice available to them at the time.

Getting What You Want

Have you ever been tempted to think that if you could just get what you wanted, you'd be happy? Whenever you decide that where you are is not where you want to be, and where you want to be is somewhere else, you will feel unhappy. Working towards making changes must be done without attachment to the outcome. Otherwise you run the danger of falling into obsession with getting results. The issue of whether you get what you want or not, becomes all-consuming. If there is uncertainty and lack of control over getting what you want, this can trigger all kinds of panic reactions. These fears are often replays of your past and have little to do with what is going on now. When you don't get what you want, the disappointment can make you angry and bitter. Ironically, even if you do get what you want, you may still be disappointed because lasting happiness does not come from getting a particular result.

The mistake begins with believing that happiness can be obtained from outside oneself. Often the old needs from childhood that have never been fulfilled are still propelling you into thinking that some new person or thing will heal this old wound. Happiness comes from love, wholeness and peace. It is an inner state of being, that comes naturally as you become more connected with who you really are, your gifts and your purpose. As long as you are fighting to get something, or trying to meet some old need, happiness will elude you. Whenever you feel disappointed, frustrated or like you're suffering a loss of some kind, it is an invitation to let go of some need or attachment.

Here's a story about someone who found a way to heal this kind of issue. A usually bright and bubbly young woman, who was recently diagnosed with MS (Multiple Sclerosis), felt frantic about her new love relationship. Although all had gone extremely well for three months, she felt something was not right. Her boyfriend talked about needing space and started creating distance between them. She became fearful that he would stop loving her, or that the magic would go, or that he would reject her. To her horror all her old betrayals came back to haunt her. As her old wounds resurfaced, she became consumed with an inner rage so great that she could hardly breathe! Her panic felt like a ball of volcanic lava swirling through her body. She found she could no longer behave normally around her boyfriend. Then she said and did things she regretted.

Her pattern of relationship problems went back a long time. Her parents had divorced when she was twenty-two. But in fact, she remembered significant fights when she was only eight years old. Seeing her mother in tears, she had decided her job was to keep the family together. Ever since that time, she had gone out of her way to do everything for everyone else. She gave her all to keep the family together. Inside her though, a rage and revenge grew about never feeling loved. The MS must have taken years to develop in her body. She wondered about the relationship between her illness and her long pattern of over-giving, sacrifice and martyrdom. Was what was happening in her current relationship, actually a re-play of all her old family wounds?

Imagining she could travel back through time, she envisaged a past life experience, just like a dream. She saw a very young boy flying a kite near an old oak tree. Meanwhile, his whole family was being murdered by burglars inside the house. When he discovered that he had lost everyone and everything, his panic and rage nearly killed him, as he could barely breathe. At first, her Heart delivered positive healing lessons to alleviate the situation: Everything happens for a reason; All is love, reason and peace; Truth is love; Under the pain is love and peace; It is possible to connect with that love and peace; He will be protected and cared for; God will look after him; He needs to trust that he is safe in God's hands.

But surprisingly an inner conflict surfaced as a new anger ignited in the character of the young boy: God had not protected them! Even worse, he felt the family had never loved him enough! Actually this revealed a deeper reason for the story.

He had created a revenge story, so he wouldn't have to succeed or show up! He could devote himself to avenging this murderous deed by being a failure in his own life.

More lessons from the Heart came through: Be in the present moment without demands or expectations; Trust, live and embrace what one has; Believe in oneself, in the power of choice. But then more inner conflict interrupted as his guilt and fear took over – he was terrified he would make bad choices and mess up again! More lessons: God is inside you; You made the choices that were right for you at the time; The ultimate goal is Love, no matter how you choose to get there.

An even deeper layer of rebelliousness intruded with disbelief. He couldn't believe any of these sweet sayings. He didn't want to be caught out. He feared being let down again! He could lose! Of course another positive payoff for losing everything and his family, was that he could never be let down again. The Heart gave more lessons: Trust, Love and believe in yourself; Understand it comes from inside so he can't betray himself; Love oneself to be able to give and receive love.

He had never trusted before and didn't know how. He felt sadness, and anger with himself for not believing. There was frustration about no one ever showing him the way. There was huge stubbornness and a desire to stay in control, because there was no belief that God would support him. This finally seemed to hit the core issue: the hurt, fear and loss of trust in God. The battle being waged was all about the illusions of trying to be in control, trying to get love, and trying to be safe. Gradually, the layers of anger, fear and inner conflict lifted and as the boy began to accept the lessons from the Heart so did the young woman.

The battle in this dream scene reflected the young woman's current relationship problem perfectly! In taking on board all the positive lessons, it was easier for her to let go of the attachment to needing love. Her energy began to flow again. As she became more willing to let go and trust, she took a new step forward spiritually. Within hours she began to rely less on outside sources for her happiness. Being more connected to her true self, she found it easier to feel love, and know what was true for her in the relationship.

Whenever you are chasing whatever it is you think will bring you happiness, you live a life of delusion, like a bad dream. Happiness is impossible there. Whenever you can let go, and trust enough to experience the moment, you experience really being alive and 'in the flow', where magical and miraculous things can happen. Happiness, peace and love are then natural and real.

> *Illusions are investments. They will last as long as you value them . . . The only way to dispel illusions is to withdraw all investment from them.*
>
> A Course in Miracles

Have you ever noticed that some people are happy having very little? In their map of reality, they have everything they need, and feel content. Their happiness is not dependent on getting something or wanting things to be different. If you were to live in their circumstances, you might have a different map, and feel discontented. Notice that the reality of the situation is the same, but because each person's perceptions, or maps, of that reality are different, they respond differently. When you or someone you know has a problem due to being attached to a certain map of reality, remember this new principle: people respond to their *maps* of reality, not to reality itself.

If you are holding on to something, or if you are attached to having things be a certain way, or if you just want something too much, take this opportunity to make a better choice. You can never know for sure what will bring you happiness. The world is full of people who have succeeded, but are still not happy. The sooner you let go, the sooner you can begin enjoying real inner peace and happiness right now. When you let go completely, you open the door to miracles in your life. What is true for you can then appear.

Exercise: Letting go ....

1. What do you believe will bring you happiness? What is currently eluding you that causes you frustration or fear?
2. What is it you really want? Maybe you are spending tons of energy trying to get it, or maybe you are feeling the frustration

or disappointment of not getting it. Identify what it is that you want.

3. Notice that this is not the same as your true Purpose. This thing you want has become like an obsession. How long have you been trying to get this, and in how many different ways?

4. What do you believe it would give you if you got it? Some form of love, approval, acceptance? Being in control? Some kind of safety, or security?

5. What feelings are associated with it?

6. Allow the feelings, about wanting this thing, to guide you on a journey going back through time to discover the origin of this. Imagine a story that would explain why this has been so important to you. Explore the metaphors of your story and write down the key points.

7. Ask your Heart for the positive lessons that can give you deeper understanding and help you let go of this obsession, and the feelings associated with it. Be thorough and find a better perspective for each key point of the story.

8. When it is appropriate, and you can let go, commit to an on-going willingness to continue to let it go whenever it might re-surface.

....

Forgiveness

When someone has made a mistake, there may be layers of blame and guilt to release. There may be someone you've never forgiven for some mistake that hurt you in the past. Sometimes the person that most needs forgiveness is you! Maybe you said or did things you feel you will never stop regretting and cringing about. How many years have you been silently pointing a finger of blame, either at yourself or someone else? Do you really want your whole life to be about this mistake? How long must the punishment last? Even criminals are released from prison for good behaviour. What do you have to gain by holding on to the guilt or blame?

Sometimes people confuse forgiveness with condoning someone else's bad behaviour. Forgiving them feels like letting them off the hook. But your bitterness and lack of forgiveness do much more to hurt you than anyone else. Just as your forgiveness can set you free. It is important to differentiate the person who made the mistake from their bad behaviour. To take a deeper, more understanding perspective of what led someone to making a mistake is always useful. It is never appropriate to condone bad behaviour.

> *Perhaps it will be helpful to remember*
> *That no one can be angry at a fact.*
> *It is always an interpretation*
> *That gives rise to negative emotions,*
> *Regardless of their seeming justification*
> *By what appears as fact.*

A Course in Miracles

What can help the forgiveness process is to imagine stepping into the other person's shoes, and imagine looking at the world through their eyes. What was their whole life like from the time they were conceived? What was their experience? What kind of parents did they have and what kind of love did they receive? What sort of beliefs, experiences and upbringing contributed to making them the way they became? When you begin to see things from their perspective, you can get a more true understanding of why they said or did the things they did. Just imagine what they must believe to be true, and what their fears are. It is not necessary to agree with what they thought, just to appreciate that they are that way.

If you have not been able to forgive yourself for some mistake, remember that you do not deserve less than other people. Often it feels easier to forgive others than to forgive yourself, because you know your own higher principles; you knew better, or you knew you were making a mistake and still did it! But if you continue to blame and punish yourself, instead of learning the lesson and moving on, you stay stuck. Not forgiving yourself means you are making yourself more special than everyone else. If only *you* deserve such punishment, and only *you* can never be forgiven, you are actually saying you are so special that no one in the universe could forgive you. It is like trying to excel at being the 'baddest' of the bad. Because it's a funny kind of arrogance and competition, it no longer has much to do with the original mistake that might have been forgiven. Make a better choice and forgive everyone, even yourself.

Forgiveness is possibly the most important step you can make towards clearing the way for your Dream Script to manifest into reality. As much as you hold on to the smallest amount of blame, guilt or revengeful thoughts, you will block the positive energy that might move you forward. Guilt keeps you stuck where you are. Whether it is your own guilt or the guilt you judge in someone else, it will not allow you to move forward. The forgiveness you feel sincerely in your own Heart will set you free. The following inner exercise does not require you to say or do anything outwardly in order to forgive another person. Real forgiveness is about how you honestly feel in your own Heart.

Exercise: Forgiveness...

Who do you most need to forgive? A Course in Miracles says that if you can truly forgive one person, ALL are forgiven.

1. Close your eyes and imagine a small dark stage in front of you and below you, with a spotlight shining down on it.
2. Invite the person you most need to forgive to step into the spotlight and have him or her look up at you. It might be someone in your life now, or from the distant past. They may have already passed away, but their memory lives on in your mind. (It could also be yourself.)
3. Imagine that there is a pale blue, grey cord connecting you, running from your belly button down to theirs. Through this hollow cord has passed all the experiences you have shared together.
4. In your mind, take this opportunity to state the facts of whatever happened that needs forgiveness. Share whatever you have been withholding.
5. Think about the lessons you have learned as a result of what has happened. Appreciate how you have grown, what qualities you have developed. Share what could have been done to rectify the situation.
6. Access a time in your life when you know you forgave someone completely. Remember what that felt like, and what you said to yourself.

7. Allow the person on the stage to say whatever they need to say to you, and just listen.

8. Take this opportunity to forgive this person to the best of your ability, from the bottom of your heart, for anything they ever said or did, or didn't say or didn't do, that hurt you. Make a promise of what you will do from now on, thanks to this experience and what you have learned.

9. Allow this person to forgive you in the same way.

10. Ask this person: 'Do you support me in all of my magnificence, in all that I've come to be and do?' Just notice their response.

11. The cord that joins you is full of the debris from the past. It is polluted with old thinking. Imagine you have a 'Golden Sword of Truth' in your hand and cut the cord, in the middle, allowing the cord to be reabsorbed back into each one of you appropriately, thereby ending the story of this misdemeanour completely.
(Should you wish to renew your relationship with this person, all you have to do – at any time you choose – is to think one unconditionally loving thought towards this person, and a new cord will spring into being.)

12. If they look distressed after the cord has been cut, call their Guardian Angel to support them, and guide them to wherever they need to go.

Once the stage is empty, you can repeat this exercise for every person you need to forgive, including yourself at whatever age you feel most guilty about.

Adapted from the Hawaiian Huna practice of Ho'o pono pono.

Forgiveness is the key to happiness. Whenever you do not forgive, you are choosing to live in judgement instead. This will never bring you peace and happiness or help to make your Dream Script a reality. So repeat the forgiveness process as many times as necessary until you have completely forgiven anyone and everyone, including yourself, for any past hurts and mistakes. How will you know when you have forgiven someone? You will be able to separate the mistaken behaviour from the person. You will feel good knowing that they are happy and thriving. You will be able to connect with their innocence, or at least be able to see the small child within them that was once innocent. You will feel at peace inside. When you can give, like you used to give before the mistake happened, you have truly forgiven. This is not about overlooking a mistake, it is about re-connecting with a deeper sense of truth and understanding. Forgiveness can clear your path to your Dream Script.

When you have finished all the exercises in this chapter, and feel that you have healed all the elements that required attention, you are ready to move on to the next step: making final adjustments to your Dream Script and aligning your energies to make it happen.

Chapter Summary
Principles:
People respond to their maps of reality, not to reality.
Let go of attachments.
Forgiveness can heal anything.

Checklist:
1. Heal the past issues
   a. Identify the feelings or beliefs that hook you to a past event story
   b. From a safe observer point of view, note how you developed certain beliefs, qualities, strengths in this story
   c. Re-evaluate, reframe, and gather new insights
2. Remember and use principles
3. Let go of obsessively wanting too much.
   a. What do you want?
   b. What past stories are associated with that?
   c. Reframe and gather positive insights
   d. Let go of the needing and wanting
4. Forgive everyone, including yourself
   a. Clear the air
   b. Forgive to the best of your ability
   c. Cut the ties to the history of blame

Aligning Your Energy

There is one thing in this world which you must never forget to do. Human beings come into this world to do particular work. That work is their purpose, and each is specific to the person. If you forget everything else and not this, there's nothing to worry about. If you remember everything else and forget your true work, then you will have done nothing in your life.

RUMI

By now, you probably appreciate the many ways your Dream Script for your life may be different from the current script you have been running. Perhaps you discovered subtle elements in your old script: hidden needs, negative feelings, or outmoded beliefs from the past that were holding you back. Maybe you've already made enormous changes in how you think and feel. Hopefully, your new understandings will continue to inspire and support you as you move forward towards your purpose and your Dream Script. You may have a much clearer idea now of who you are and what is true for you.

Looking at the Dream Script for your life that you wrote in Chapter 1, how much more possible does it seem? Are there any aspects that you need to adjust? If you are more capable of achieving this now, does it start to feel even more exciting? You may find that you are ready to take the first steps towards bringing your Dream Script into reality. Maybe it's time to prepare some plans of action. How much do you feel you deserve to have this Dream Script? Does all of you want this script, or do you have some internal voices pushing you in another direction? Do you have any inner conflict going on? If your mind is being torn in different directions, your energy cannot flow smoothly towards creating your Dream Script. Inner conflicts pull you off centre, away from your purpose and what is true for you. In order to create a smooth pathway for your Dream Script to become a reality, it is important to bring all your energy into alignment.

You might not even be aware that you have an inner conflict. Particularly if you are a positive, proactive type of person, you probably spend so much time moving forward, that it takes you by surprise when something obstructs your progress – especially if it comes from within. You only become aware of an inner conflict when everything grinds to a halt and you are left wondering what is going on. It can take some practice to become aware of inner feelings that disagree with your plans.

On the other hand, you may be a person who is only too aware that you have a chatter box of internal voices telling you what to do and what not to do, criticising, judging, warning, coaxing and cajoling you. Whenever you try to make a decision, a battle begins. No matter which direction you take, only part of your energy goes into it. The rest still wants to go in the opposite direction! If you find making decisions difficult, it's probably because you have not known how to resolve your inner conflicts. Or maybe you make decisions, but never follow through with them. The following story may give you some ideas about how to deal with internal conflicts.

A very experienced business consultant had finally concluded a long and intense, eighteen-month project. The job had gone well, but included giving out inevitable redundancies. He was so good at delivering these that he was known as the 'axe man'. But he was well liked because he did his best to protect the team, and was very fair and respectful to everyone. Now that most of this role was complete, he felt spent. His batteries were flat. However, the management didn't want him to leave. They enjoyed his lively debates and loved to argue with him. He was the management's safety net. Without him there, it felt like something important was missing.

So they negotiated a new role for him, as a Coach and Mentor to the management team. He looked forward to stepping forward in this completely new capacity. To his surprise, however, as soon as he stepped back into the building, he found that his old role was almost impossible to escape. He felt drawn back to protecting his old team. They were equally delighted to see him, thinking they could have him back to make all their decisions again. But he didn't want to be the Project Director anymore! He wanted to be a facilitator rather than a director. He described it as leaving his old 'axe man' role, to do more of the 'pink, fluffy stuff'. But the 'axe man' energy and passion felt much more comfortable compared to what he dismissively called the 'pink, fluffy stuff'!

He obviously felt some conflict about what he really wanted his role to be. Would he miss the stimulus from the 'axe man' role? He said that he could get that sort of stimulus elsewhere with other companies he worked for. Would he be happy doing only 'pink fluffy stuff' during one meeting a week? He was very clear that both roles satisfied his highest objectives and purpose. It seemed that it was only a matter of behavioural style, how he chose to deliver those objectives. So I began to wonder if the conflict was in the metaphors he chose to describe them.

I asked him what the 'axe man' thought of the 'pink, fluffy' number. The answer was full of disdain, describing it as weak and ineffectual. The 'axe man' valued strength, directness, protection and respect, no bullshit. We then explored a more true sense of value for the 'pink, fluffy' number. As he accessed the useful qualities of rapport, relationship, and agility, it became clear that these were aspects of his untapped feminine side. He admitted that only recently, thanks to learning to dance with his wife, he had begun to appreciate the value of relationship. Suddenly his 'pink fluffy' metaphor spontaneously changed into a dancer! Meanwhile, as the masculine 'axe man' listened, he also went through a metamorphosis, becoming a Buddhist monk (still with an axe), who directed his strength without violence and who stayed attuned to his core principles.

We negotiated between the dancer and the monk to help them appreciate each other's talents and positive qualities until we reached a place of so much compatibility that they could work together easily. His metaphors again spontaneously changed to reflect this at the end. The dancer became a gymnast who moved with precision and elegance, while the axe man no longer needed any armour. He felt much more comfortable and congruent with whichever role he chose to play, using whichever behaviour would serve the purpose in the moment.

He who knows others is wise;
He who knows himself is enlightened.

Lao–Tzu

There are several factors which seem to help in dealing with inner conflicts. First, it's important to listen to the metaphors that are naturally used to describe the different parts. Remember that your unconscious mind loves to play with metaphors. Whenever you use symbols, stories and metaphors, you are more likely to access the deeper parts of your mind where the problems need to be solved. Take the metaphors seriously, and work with them playfully. Each symbol may express a great deal of information. A picture is worth a thousand words. Allow these images to change and evolve and flow.

Another important element is to elicit fully the intentions and goals of each part. Appreciate the feelings being expressed. Honour the desires, no matter how destructive they may seem at first. Remember that behind every behaviour there is a positive intention. Stay curious to discover ALL the intentions a part might want for you. When you truly understand each part, and appreciate all the different qualities and gifts each one holds for you, it will be easy to negotiate co-operation and integration.

Exercise: Inner conflicts ....

1. As you think about your ideal script, do you feel any resistance towards believing it is possible and desirable? Are there any voices of dissent?
2. Welcome these voices or feelings, especially if they sound cynical or derogatory. These represent your integrity in some way and need to be honoured. Find out what is wanted, and appreciate the good qualities that are intended.
3. Notice that it takes at least two sides to make a conflict, so take note of the qualities of each side and what each one wants for you.

4. What judgements do they have about each other? It might help to separate them physically by imagining you could sit them on two different chairs. Let each one speak and air its judgements about the other.
5. Explore each one fully, noting any metaphors that appear to be associated with them. What does each one want for you? And if it got that, what would that give you? Continue asking that question until you get a full understanding of each part.
6. Hopefully, you will discover some common ground, some basis for the two of them beginning to respect each other better, and more willingness to communicate and work together.
7. Keep negotiating between the two until they feel happier to integrate their different natures and bring a more balanced sense of wholeness to you.

When you are alone, centred, meditative and quiet, you are less likely to be aware of any internal conflict. Sometimes the more hidden feelings only surface with the friction of rubbing against other people and events. So when you are being still, peaceful and calm, and things are not happening the way you want them in your life, consider that to be a sign that there could be a hidden conflict under that quiet surface.

It is much easier to notice internal conflict when it creates craziness inside your head. Internal dialogue can drive you nuts, keep you awake all night and make you worried and stressed all day. But by listening to what each voice needs to express, and by respecting the higher purpose of each part, you can turn even the worst internal battles into reasonable discussions and reach agreement. Then you can enjoy a whole new level of still, quiet spiritual space.

Are you aware that you think more than 40,000 different thoughts every day? Unfortunately, they are probably the same 40,000 thoughts that you thought yesterday and the day before! Our brains keep re-treading the same paths again and again. Have you noticed that not only do you have those thoughts, but you also have thoughts and feelings about your thoughts?

Without even consciously knowing what you are thinking, your feelings react to whatever your brain is thinking about. You might like some of your thoughts, but dislike others. Sometimes you may feel angry, ashamed or frightened about your thoughts, so you try to delete them or control them. A critical voice starts telling you what you should and shouldn't do, think or feel. 'Don't be so stupid! You shouldn't have said that! Why aren't you more loving!' And then other voices chime in with strategies to fix it: 'You should be nice to people. Don't be sad! You need to prove how good you are.' And then rebellious voices start fighting against the helpful suggestions, and once again the craziness takes over. It is not surprising that many people would like to push this internal dialogue down out of their awareness. After you have dealt with the most important inner conflicts, there is another way to handle these inner voices.

You can learn how to 'contain' the craziness in a loving way, where it no longer runs your behaviour. A surprisingly effective way to achieve this, is to give yourself permission to feel, think and experience whatever is going on. So, for example, say to yourself: 'It's OK to say "NO" without feeling guilty. It's OK to feel insecure, out of control and still be in control. It's OK to feel scared and still love people'. Just saying this, gives you time to pause, and release some of the tension. When you give yourself permission to be the way you are, you can just get on with life, content with knowing that your mind will always be deviant! But this acceptance will create a better relationship with your feelings that allows you to enjoy the present moment, and just be real. From here, choice and real change are possible.

I have lived on the lip
Of insanity, wanting to know reasons,
Knocking on a door. It opens.
I've been knocking from the inside!

Rumi

Experiment by practising this compassionate way of being with your inner self. The more you use this way of listening to your mind, and just being with the energy, the more your unconscious mind will begin to trust you, and work with you rather than against you. This is a way to love and honour the different voices of your mind, instead of resisting them, denying them, or trying to delete them from your awareness. Give them freedom of speech!

Exercise: Dealing with internal dialogue.............................

1. First listen to your disruptive internal dialogue, maybe even noting down some of the craziness. What are the 'shoulds', 'shouldn'ts', 'dos' and 'don'ts'? If it is about someone else, notice how, when and where you are doing the similar things. You only notice their behaviour because it is familiar. Commit to staying in awareness, and notice your inner thoughts.
2. What feelings are generated as a result of this internal dialogue?
3. Imagine you can hold all of these thoughts and feelings in a compassionate, non-judgemental way. Take your awareness down to your Heart and allow your Heart to assist you in answering the questions below.
4. Give yourself permission to have each of these thoughts and feelings, but convert each one from criticism to permission, for example:
   I'll never make it!
   It's OK for me to make it and I am making it.
   It's OK for me to never make it and still be a good person.
   Don't be lazy!
   It's OK for me to be lazy and still get things done.
   It's OK for me to be active.
   It's OK for me to take my time and stay focused.
   You're not good enough!
   It's OK for me to be good enough and I am.
   It's OK for me to be not good enough and still like myself.
   It's OK for people to think I'm not good enough and still be good enough.
5. Keep asking yourself open questions relevant to your own negative judgements e.g.: It's OK for me to . . . Just pause and wait for your Heart's answer. Keep asking until all of your negative feelings dissolve and you feel more at peace.
6. You can use this process every day to honour and clear

your emotional state. Sometimes the old feelings come back – just give yourself more permission. Occasionally you might get a metaphorical answer – some action you would never want to enact. Just ask what does this permission stand for? What inner experience would be achieved if I did do that? Again wait for the inner answer. When the energy of the voices diminishes, you are finished for the moment.

7. Reminder: If you are in a situation where these voices intrude, distract or annoy you, you can put them on temporary 'hold' by just turning the volume down, or putting a filter on the voice to make it sound like a cartoon character, or a sexy movie star. Sometimes it can also help to move the location of the voice – for example, let it speak from your left elbow or your right big toe. Not quite the same, is it?

Process adapted from Swami Anantananda
Example: One client had internal dialogue about 'Don't mess up!' and 'I look ugly and unlovable.' This unhelpful voice came up every time she was on a date, destroying her self confidence. She then had to be very careful with every word she said, and everything she did. No matter how great she looked, she never got to feel beautiful. Instead she waited for criticism, frightened of being rejected. Her main feeling was fear, which was not attractive. So she took her awareness to her heart centre and started making statements of permission, and letting the Heart fill in the blanks. 'It's OK for me to mess up . . . and I'll still be lovable if I do. It's OK for me to be ugly . . . and still be lovable. It's OK for me to be unlovable . . . to others, and still love myself. It's OK for me to make mistakes . . . and still give my love to others. It's OK to look however I look . . . and still love myself. She used these new statements like a mantra, repeating them to herself and found she started to feel more open and playful.

After you get good at doing this, a sure sign of your expertise will be that you start taking yourself more lightly. When you stop and listen to all the crazy thoughts that go on inside your head every day, it is much harder to take any of them so seriously.

Giving yourself permission to be the way you are allows you to accept reality instead of resisting it. Then you can have full access to your true qualities and be more balanced. The fear expressed through internal dialogue cannot be the whole truth about you. When you are willing to laughingly admit to yourself that your thoughts are not always rational, logical or even that intelligent, you can begin to channel the power of your mind more effectively to listen to your Heart.

> *What does the Zen monk say to the hot dog stand vendor?*
> *'Make me one with everything!'*
>
> *What does the vendor say when the monk asks for change*
> *from a £20 note?*
> *'Change comes from within!'*

Making Choices

Making choices is possibly the most precious and most important gift we have. Changing your thinking, and making a better choice, a choice that is more aligned with your Heart, can transform the most difficult situations. When you are completely in tune with your purpose, your giftedness, and what is true for you, making choices becomes simple. Often there is only one easy choice.

When other people or events seem to govern your behaviour, it feels like you have no choice. If you 'have to' or 'should' do things to please someone else's rules or requirements, don't you feel resentful? Even if you agree with those rules, you might inwardly rebel against the sense of being controlled. Oddly, you may be perfectly happy to perform a certain action, but the fact someone asked you to do it takes away all the pleasure and enjoyment. Most people prefer to be free to make their own choices even if it means they have to suffer their own mistakes. By writing your Dream Script, you have already re-connected with your inner desires. And by exploring the various aspects of your current script, you've had the opportunity to resolve several issues that may have been holding you back. The next step is to re-write your

Dream Script, so that your inner choices set a true direction for your life.

Setting a Direction

There is an important difference between setting a goal and having a direction. Many people do neither, and wonder why their lives seem to flounder. Those who do neither will benefit greatly from learning simple goal setting procedures. But when you become adept at setting goals, you might fall into the trap of always striving to achieve something. If you are a hard taskmaster on yourself or others, you might be wise to learn how to do things the easy way. The value of having a direction instead of trying to achieve goals is well illustrated in the following story.

Expert coach, Michael Neill, wrote about an interview with Admiral James Stockdale, who was the highest ranking United States military officer held in a prisoner of war camp during the Vietnam war. For eight years, he was kept primarily in isolation and tortured in a prison with conditions so brutal it became ironically known as 'the Hanoi Hilton'.

Under these intense and relentless circumstances, Stockdale developed his reputation as a leader, an innovator, and a man with unbreakable character. Many of his fellow POWs credit his influence and example as one of the key factors in their own ability to persevere through otherwise insufferable conditions.

When asked how he managed to stay sane and strong under such brutal conditions, Admiral Stockdale said: 'I never lost faith in the end of the story. I never doubted not only that I would get out, but also that I would prevail in the end and turn the experience into the defining event of my life, which, in retrospect, I would not trade.'

When asked the difference between the men who made it and the ones who did not survive, his answer was surprising: 'We had a name for the people who weren't going to make it out,' Stockdale said. 'We called them "the optimists". They were the ones who said, "We're going to be out by Christmas." And Christmas would come, and Christmas would go. Then they'd say, "We're going to be out by Easter." And Easter would come, and Easter would go. And then Thanksgiving, and then it would be Christmas again. And they died of a broken heart.'

Determining your direction will sustain you with the faith and perseverance necessary to keep you moving forward on your true path. Setting goals is very useful, but not as powerful. If you achieve your goals, it might spur you onwards with optimism, but if you fail, your disappointment may discourage you completely. Being guided by your true direction, will help you succeed regardless of difficulties. When you face impossible challenges, and terrible traumas, your direction can give you an inner strength that is invincible. Tell yourself that you will prevail in the end, no matter what may be happening now. What can help you do this, is to consider the larger perspective. Who else will benefit, how will the world be a better place, or what wisdom will grow and develop in your character?

When we quit thinking primarily about ourselves and our own self preservation, we undergo a truly heroic transformation of consciousness.

Joseph Campbell

Common coaching advice recommends setting achievable goals. Smaller objectives or outcomes, that can be easily measured, are considered safer because that avoids the danger of taking on too much. The theory is that if you set your goals too high, you might over-promise and under-deliver. The result might end in discouragement, shame and self-loathing. This kind of goal setting is good advice if you are at the stage of planning your first steps towards a known outcome.

Having a direction is not about setting goals at all. Your direction is more of an inner life purpose, a soul purpose, or a spiritual purpose. It is not so much about what you do as it is about who you are, why you are here, and what meaning you would like your life to have. Discovering your direction requires an intuitive sense of being connected with your Heart. You may already know your direction, or you may enjoy allowing it to be revealed to you over the rest of your life. The man in the next story had been so good at achieving his goals, that it really surprised him to feel at loss. He needed to discover his direction.

A space scientist fell into such deep depression that he had to leave work for three weeks. Although he used to enjoy everything he did, he no longer found his work challenging. He didn't want to do it for twenty more years! He thought there must be more to life than work and spending money. What puzzled him was that he had actually achieved his childhood dream: designing space missions for NASA. But now that he had done that, he didn't know what to do next! He didn't have any goals to aim for. Being a forward-looking man who always succeeded in achieving his outcomes, this situation puzzled him and made him feel out of control.

Despite having fulfilled his childhood dream, he had never felt genuinely successful. His parents had always made him feel like he should have done better, no matter how well he did. Consequently he had developed a tendency to look at the negative side of things: the glass being half empty. Until this depression, he had never been aware of his feelings. Looking back, it seemed like his life had always been happy before. In fact, what he used to consider happiness was an unfeeling state of independence. Now he found it surprisingly easy to burst into tears. His emotions would swing up and down from rage to sadness, with a cacophony of voices interrupting each other inside his head. His usual clarity of thought had vanished and his brain felt like it was about to blow up.

He described his life: it felt like he had been going down a road with very high hedges on either side. He had never seen the sky, or the fields, or the other paths he could have taken. Now, when he dreamed of being more spontaneous and making changes, he felt scared, out of control, overwhelmed and unable to cope. Inside his head, one frustrated voice kept urging him to just 'GO! Get away! Get a Life!' But another voice kept saying, 'You shouldn't do that! Be sensible! You have to pay the mortgage!' The internal battle resulted in complete inertia.

We opened communication between these two voices. The sensible one seemed to live in his head and felt like a wagging finger, always telling him what he should and shouldn't do. It believed that a stiff upper lip was the best policy, and had no tolerance for irrational emotions! The other frustrated voice that just wanted to get away and escape, lived in his throat area, and was more connected to his Heart and feelings. Neither one believed that the other was worth listening to, and neither one trusted the other.

After some careful negotiating, it became clear that what both parts wanted was actually very similar: peace, quiet, being at ease, having 'a life'. But the emotional one was afraid of being controlled by the sensible one. While the sensible one was terrified of being overwhelmed by those irrational feelings. Gradually through more communication and reframing, they began to relax and trust each other, until he finally reached a place where he could be anywhere on the feelings scale of sad to happy, and still be OK. Here at last he found freedom. He was able then to release some very old stale feelings and discover a new sense of oneness.

As he intuitively brought the integrated parts deep into his centre, he began to feel more balanced. From this centre, he could begin to trust his ability to feel what was right for him, and move with more certainty of direction. Now that his attitude felt so different, he was relieved to think it might not be necessary to make drastic changes. His eyes brightened and he looked lighter and relieved as he talked about feeling more connected: he suddenly felt he was a part of something bigger than himself. To 'get a life' now meant enjoying everything he had. From this attitude of gratitude, he could move in any direction he chose.

The question, 'What do you want?' must be answered.
You are answering it every minute and every second,
And each moment of decision is a judgement
That is anything but ineffectual.
Its effects will follow automatically until the decision is changed.

A Course in Miracles

If you have times when you don't know what you want, don't despair. Instead of just jumping at the first idea that enters your head, allow yourself to have some space and time. Wait for the right path to show itself. Clear the way by removing any hidden conflicts. By all means, explore lots of different directions, but stay connected to your Heart and purpose. Ask your Heart to tell you which roads to traverse and which ones to avoid. It may be the right time to re-think your Dream Script. Are there adjustments that need to be made? Perhaps you now have the courage to think even bigger than before. Maybe there are things you want to add or clarify.

Exercise: Re-write your Dream Script..................................

1. Take a really objective view of your Dream Script now. What would you like to adjust? What conscious and unconscious goals need to be met? Take some time to re-view your script now.
2. Is there anything that stops you from changing your course or setting goals that are different from your current script?
3. Are there any conflicting feelings, ideas or judgements that need to be sorted out?
4. Have you resolved any issues about *not* having your Dream Script? Have you no more excuses, no more avoidance, no more payoffs for not living it?
5. How can your new Dream Script become the most motivating, compelling direction for you? How does it already inspire you?

....

Being Too Busy

Some people have been such good achievers their lives are too full. Does this describe you? Do you have so much to do, that you are constantly juggling, rushing around and striving to keep up with impossible schedules? Are you so busy that you find it difficult to relax? You know you are in trouble when you can't slow down long enough to really enjoy anything. Are you so focused on getting what you want, and so stressed that you haven't had time to notice whether you are happy or not? You might have fallen into that trap of thinking that when you have achieved a particular goal, or after you have acquired a particular thing, only then can you relax and be happy. Chasing after goals in this way, will certainly keep you busy, but are you moving in alignment with your true direction?

Perhaps you think that you should be that busy. Do you think being busy equals being productive? Do you believe that if you worked even harder, then you would be successful and happy? What happens if you don't enjoy working that hard? In fact, a possible downside of your new Dream Script could be that it might require too much effort! If it looks like too much hard work, somehow you might never get around to it. But procrastination would only be a sign that you need to go back and check for hidden needs. When you've created a Dream Script that is truly aligned with your direction and purpose, it will feel almost effortless. Any work involved will feel like fun because you enjoy it so much. The motivation comes naturally. Instead of chasing after material things to make you feel good, or to compensate hours of doing something you loathe, you'll just surprise yourself with your dedication.

It is preoccupation with possessions, more than anything else, that prevents us from living freely and nobly.

Bertrand Russell

The media bombards us constantly with images and promises of how happy we will be if we buy this product, how sexy we will be if we use this perfume, how successful we will look if we drive this car. But advertising didn't create this trend of living such busy lives and being so driven. Advertising only hooks your internal beliefs about striving for achievement. When you believe that achieving something, or having more 'stuff', looking perfect, or proving something will bring you happiness and fulfilment, it can cause trouble. Oddly enough, it can even cause problems if you succeed in having it all, as the following example shows.

A highly successful career woman had it all: fantastic job, loving husband, two great kids, perfect home, nanny, cars, toys, holidays. Being extremely intelligent and competent, she managed to keep everything organised perfectly, but her husband complained about her being too controlling. In fact, she never stopped long enough to take a breath. Eventually, her stress levels had built up to such a degree that she felt like she was in a cyclone.

While her house was being redecorated, with the furniture stacked up in some rooms, the usual perfection of her home became a mess. Then she decided to do a de-tox diet programme, which unwittingly triggered her old bulimia pattern. She noticed that she was becoming more obsessive and perfectionist than usual. With her stress levels running so high, it would take very little to push her over the edge. Feeling miserable and crying a lot, she became frightened that she might have another bout of depression and have to take Prozac again.

She wished she could be more like her laid-back husband, who could just 'Be'. She longed to be able to just sit down and enjoy a glass of wine. Why couldn't she get pleasure out of simple sensory things instead of everything having to look so perfect? In her map of the world, everything was judged by appearances and what she achieved. Being extraordinarily disciplined, she was a super achiever. Anything she decided to do, she did, and did well. But she knew from personal experience, after ten years being bulimic, that being thin doesn't make you happy. She also knew that striving for excellence in a super career only makes you stressed, and that having money doesn't bring happiness either. When her children were away for the weekend, the house was perfectly tidy, and she had no pressing work – she didn't know what to do! She could not rest, didn't feel happy, and then felt angry because she wasn't busy!

She wanted to be perfect. She needed everything to be 'just so'. When she said she was going to do something, like go to the gym, she had to go, or it would cause huge mental distress until she did. When I asked her what achieving all these things would bring her, she answered, 'people will approve of me and love me for being perfect'. She believed she had to earn love, and if she didn't perform well enough, she felt panic.

Of course, she knew exactly where this had come from. Her father, a successful and disciplined professional, had ruled her upbringing with cruel demands for perfect behaviour. When her room was untidy, her favourite possessions were flushed down the toilet. He told her she was a 'disappointment' when she couldn't remember her nine times table, and made it clear that she was only worthy of love if she performed well. His parents had raised him in a similar way, during the Second

World War. His parents had never been able to show love or affection to their only child. He must have grown up believing that perfection earned approval. Later he married a woman he could mould and control. Their home was always picture perfect, and their children also became extensions of his need for perfection.

Her father had never ever allowed her to 'just be'. In fact, she wouldn't know who she was, if she could 'just be'. Love had always been conditional on achievement. She felt extremely angry about how much his demands upset her peace of mind. She was frightened that she might mess up her own children in the same way. When I pointed out to her that her father had also taught her to have the discipline, determination and courage to be as successful as she was, she had to admit that all the good things she had achieved were worthwhile. She liked having all those things, and she liked everything looking perfect. Therefore his input was not all bad.

Gradually, she began to appreciate that he could not help being the way he was, because of his own upbringing. As part of her process, she received positive advice from her Heart about lightening up: having a bit more fun, knowing that you are fine the way you are, that you can take the path that life opens up for you instead of controlling everything, that you can just 'be yourself', be kind, funny, caring, generous, you can stop trying so hard, get a life, and do what you really want to do. As she wished these qualities for her father, she also began to re-programme her own mind. It wasn't easy, but she even began to forgive her father.

Whether you run successful strategies of achievement, or less satisfying strategies of guilt (for not running successful strategies of achievement), your ability to feel happy and fulfilled requires an inner shift of awareness. Remembering who you are, being more present in the moment instead of planning the future, knowing you are OK no matter what is happening, and staying tuned into what is true for you, are more important than what you achieve, or don't achieve. You may already have many of the elements you want in your Dream Script. Maybe you just need to let go of overachieving long enough to enjoy what you have and who you are.

Healing does not come from anyone else.
You must accept guidance from within.

A Course in Miracles

Success and Failure

The fear of failure often causes different kinds of obsessive behaviour. If you are successfully motivated away from failure, you may get caught up in striving and over achieving as compensations. But if you feel like a total failure, and believe that nothing you do will work, then there is no motivation, just giving up and hiding. Some people are so afraid of failing that they can't even get started on a project. A principle that really helps here is: There's no such thing as failure, only feedback.

There's no such thing as failure because you learn from every experience you have in life. The feedback that you get from your experience tells you immediately what doesn't work! You don't have to make that mistake again. Have you ever noticed that you learn more from making mistakes than from doing something right the first time? Maybe you should make as many mistakes as you can! Celebrate every time you make a mistake – you have learned something! There's no failure because all it means is that you haven't achieved that result *yet*. Maybe the feedback will tell you what needs to be changed, or maybe that it wasn't even the right outcome to start with. If you are obsessed with achievement, or feeling like the world's worst failure, ask yourself the questions in the next exercise.

Exercise: Driven to success or failure? ....

Are you driving yourself too hard? Are you pushing yourself to achieve, succeed, excel? Are you planning so much for the future that you never enjoy the present? Or quite the opposite?

1. Take a long cool perspective on your life? How well are you balancing work and play? Do you find it easy to switch off and relax? What are your stress levels like?
2. If you are spending too much time striving to achieve things, ask yourself exactly what it is you hope will happen as a result of your imagined success? What are you trying to get?

3. Take another step back, and carefully, honestly assess whether the result you want is, in fact, directly linked to the activity. Will achieving this result actually give you what you want?

4. What is the cost of pushing yourself so hard? Who or what is suffering? Your health? Your family? Your colleagues? Your joie de vivre?

5. Will these achievements matter to you when you are ninety-nine years old? When you look back and re-assess your life, what will be most valuable to you, what will you feel most happy and proud about?

6. In what are other ways can you achieve what you truly want? Do you already have that? Can you just become more aware and grateful for it?

7. What can you do to help to reduce your stress levels right now – even if it was just letting go of some of the need to achieve?

....

When you feel you have completed all the exercises thoroughly enough, and made whatever changes and improvements were needed in your Dream Script, you are ready to start the manifesting process. Now you should also be more aligned with what you want, instead of being pulled in different directions internally. In fact, if you are beginning to feel like your Dream Script is not so important anymore – that's great!

Peace is an attribute IN you,
You cannot find it outside.

A Course in Miracles

Because of all the inner work you have completed so far, you should be feeling much more balanced. Knowing your gifts, your purpose, and gaining so much understanding about the hidden intentions that were operating before, all help you have a better sense of who you are and who you came to be. If you have also healed some old stories and forgiven past events and people who hurt you, then a true peacefulness cannot be far away. It is this inner state of being centred, peaceful, calm and open to receive that will allow you to begin manifesting your Dream Script almost effortlessly.

Chapter Summary:

Principle:
There is no such thing as failure, only feedback

Checklist:
1. How much more possible is your script now?
2. Is there any inner conflict about living your script?
   a. Elicit the positive intentions of each side of the conflict
   b. Negotiate a respectful way of them working together
3. Give yourself permission
   a. Reframe your internal dialogue
   b. Give yourself permission to have each thought
4. Re-write your Dream Script: set a new direction
5. Avoid the trap of being 'driven'
   a. Re-assess what you hope to get as a result of working so hard
   b. What is the cost, and what do you truly want

8

Manifesting Miracles

*What lies behind us and lies before us are small matters
compared to what lies within us. And when we bring what
is within us out into the world, miracles happen.*

H. D. THOREAU

It is time to start making miracles happen! Are you happy with
and inspired by the Dream Script you have created? Have you
been able to let go of wanting it too much or having it be a
certain way? Do you feel more connected with your giftedness,
and your purpose? Are you ready to take full responsibility for
directing your Script? Do you think you have healed all of the
important issues that used to hold you back? Are you feeling
innocent, deserving and courageous? Soon you'll be able to
know how well you've done by watching the results manifest
in your life.

The *Oxford English Dictionary* defines a miracle as 'a
remarkable and welcome event that seems impossible to explain
by means of the known laws of nature and which is therefore
attributed to a super-natural agency'. But what happens just
BEFORE a miracle takes place? Usually there is a change of
thought, or a shift in belief that is truly profound and all per-
vasive. Perhaps that is the real miracle! When you fully believe
that you can do something, when all of your thoughts are aligned,
when there is no internal conflict inside you, then you can keep
stepping forward towards what is true for you. Your inner sense
of direction will guide you around obstacles, and your inspiration will give you the patience to persevere for as long as it
takes. It is almost like being invincible. The best part though,
is that as you begin living your Dream Script, you can enjoy

every moment of it, knowing that every thing that happens is a crucial part of your journey in the story. You may even discover that you take enormous pleasure in seeing how quickly you can make positive meanings out of events you used to classify as disasters.

You'll know when you are well on the way to success when:

- You just love doing what you are doing for the sake of doing it
- Every event is an amazing adventure, no matter how small
- You welcome each challenge, and look forward to learning
- You know that every problem hides a gift
- You are curious about what you can give to everyone you meet
- You've forgotten about your Dream Script!

Of course, this requires you to continue to use many of the processes you have learned so far. Every moment of every day presents you with all kinds of choices about how you will behave, what you choose to think, and how you feel. You can use your Dream Script to guide you. Imagine how the star of your script would behave, think and feel in any particular situation. How can you turn this into an opportunity to give your gifts, and to demonstrate your purpose?

There is an old Cherokee story about a tribal elder who is teaching his grandson about life.

'A fight is going on inside me,' he said to the boy. 'It is a terrible fight and it is between two wolves.

One is evil – he is anger, envy, sorrow, regret, greed, arrogance, self-pity, guilt, resentment, inferiority, lies, false pride, superiority, and ego.

The other is good – he is joy, peace, love, hope, serenity, humility, kindness, benevolence, empathy, generosity, truth, compassion, and faith. This same fight is going on inside you – and inside every other person, too.'

The grandson thought about it for a minute and then asked his grandfather, 'Which wolf will win?'

The old Cherokee simply replied, 'The one you feed.'

In fact, your choices are much more simple than you might think. In *A Course in Miracles* it says that 'every decision is a choice between love and fear.' You are either making a choice for love, when your Dream Script is aligned with your Heart, or you are being tempted back into old patterns of fear from the past. There is no objective middle ground. What is not a form of love, is a derivative of fear. Remembering this can help you to identify which path to choose whenever you reach a fork in the road. All you need to do is listen to your Heart.

Doubt

If your Dream Script includes a BIG ambition or something that feels out of reach, you may discover some wee doubts lurking in the back of your mind. Or you might find that, despite completing all the exercises, somehow you just can't get yourself to take action and go for it. Doubt produces hesitation. It might seem more intelligent to remain uncertain until something is proved. But in fact, doubt is based on disbelief – the exact opposite of the energy you need to manifest your script into reality. Once you allow doubt to step in, your thoughts will feed the wrong wolf. Doubt is like sticking a wedge in a doorway. Although it opens the door just a little, what squeezes in quickly right behind it? All your negative judgements, criticisms, fears and other negative emotions rush in. If you don't stop the process, before you know what has happened, your mind will be directed far away from the positive energies of your Dream Script, far from your purpose, your gifts and what is true for you. What you need instead of doubt is trust.

Life is either a daring adventure, or nothing.

Helen Keller

Since it is a good idea to reframe everything to find the positive intention, surely doubt deserves that too. A positive intention for doubt might be to double check and make sure that your script is truly 'ecological'. That is, it won't cause you harm, or hurt anyone else in the environment of your life. Think carefully about the repercussions of living your Dream Script and whether it will be a good thing to have in this world. Some people worry about whether what they are asking for is true for them to have. What if it isn't 'God's plan' that this should happen? Well, if it isn't true for you, it simply won't happen! But how will you know how far you could have gone, how will you know how much you could have achieved if you don't put everything you've got into making it happen? The universe is abundant, and possibilities abound. Don't you owe it to yourself to stretch as far as you can and be the best you can be? Surely it can't be true for you to hold yourself back and stay small. Even if there are limits to what you can have or do, how do you know how far you can push those limits unless you give your best? Here is a process to help you put your doubts to rest.

Exercise: Dealing with doubt..

1. First do a reality check: Is this Dream Script possible? Do you want to do it or is it just a fantasy that you run? What would your life be like if you did live it? How would it affect other people who are important to you? What would the long-term consequences of achieving this be? (if it is something that you genuinely want to accomplish, then continue)
2. What are the doubts about taking action? Can you get in touch with the part of you that resists? Get to know this part, talk to it, and get a sense of what its concerns are. It probably has your best interests at heart. What does it fear? What is it protecting? It may think that you are being rash, or the risks are too high. Listen carefully and note down what these concerns are.
3. When or where did this behaviour originate? Has there always been a part of you that performs this function? Does being doubtful run in your family?
4. From all your present wisdom, and drawing on any insights you may receive, how differently could you think about whatever you doubt? What does your Heart have to say about this?
5. If you're ready to take action, then go for it! Make a realistic plan of action, and think of all the people you could contact for help. Brainstorm where you could get the resources you need to make this Dream Script a total success!

Dodge was a person who never had a problem with doubt. He was only nineteen when he started creating his Dream Script during a *Compassionate Coaching* training seminar. He knew exactly what he wanted: a pad in Chelsea by the time he was twenty-five, a place on a national rugby team, a Porsche, a passive income, to travel the world, have a great girlfriend and be happy. He also knew what he didn't want: he never wanted to have to work in a job for someone else, and he wasn't interested in lots of education. Although he had plenty of confidence, he wasn't sure he'd succeed in making his dreams come true. Everyone told him his talent for rugby playing was amazing, but that was no guarantee he would make a national team. What really made him stand out was his sheer determination to follow his direction. He truly followed his heart and always loved everything he was doing. As a teenager, he had fun making pocket money by selling t-shirts, sunglasses and other items to all his friends. He said he could only sell something if he believed it was really good, but he also instinctively knew what people wanted. Funnily enough, he developed a natural talent for charming people into buying his goods.

Only two years later, he found himself at Loughborough Sports University doing a degree in Sports Science and playing professional rugby for the Leicester Tigers. He felt he had landed in heaven! The pay was good and a sports car was part of the package. He thought life couldn't be better! He travelled the world playing rugby and spent six months in New Zealand. Then after playing rugby for another year with the Rugby Lions, he decided he wanted to do something different. As much as he loved rugby, he couldn't do it forever, or make the money he really wanted to make.

After getting his Sports Science degree at twenty-four, he decided to start his own business. The movie *The Full Monty* was popular then, so he talked four of his rugby chums into donning costumes and learning some choreography to perform a similar act in nightclubs. Then he also organised some playboy strippers to be part of the show. In no time at all, he talked some top nightclubs into buying his new production. His natural talent for knowing what people want made him extremely astute at designing exactly the type of entertainment that would sell.

His first event was so successful, he went on to set up a proper business. Currently his business promotes popular events at ten different nightclubs every night of the week giving him the passive income he had always dreamed of. He loves the freedom this gives him, and enjoys taking the risks. He never misses an opportunity and cannily invests his money in property where it will most probably fund his next project. So he got his pad in Chelsea, but decided to buy a Mercedes instead of a Porsche. Being incredibly handsome, charming and super successful at only twenty-seven, he confessed that having girlfriends was not a problem.

Dodge loves having the freedom to do whatever he wants, whenever he wants. Although he does work hard, he takes seven holidays a year and enjoys sharing his happiness with others. He is convinced that learning how to focus on his goals and trust they would happen were the key elements that helped him make his dreams come true.

> *In the long run, we shape our lives and we shape ourselves. The process never ends until we die. And the choices we make are ultimately our own responsibility.*
>
> Eleanor Roosevelt

If you have one main Dream Script that incorporates many goals, it may satisfy all the different areas of your life until the end of your days. However, you might find that after your Dream Script becomes a reality, you will want to repeat the process and manifest something new – a whole new direction! People live long enough now to fit in several careers and many life changes. As you change and grow, your purpose and direction might evolve and take a slightly different path. Success breeds more success, as well as more confidence to think even bigger. Using the skills you have learned in this book can continue to help you wherever your journey goes.

If you haven't already, why not stretch yourself to think beyond what you might want for yourself, and include in your Script what you might want for the world. How could your Script contribute to a much bigger plan? If you wanted to be a part of making big changes, think how motivating that would be? What if you knew that your Script would not only bring you happiness, but also benefit the world in some major way? Your energy could become so magnetic that you would attract whatever you needed to make it happen.

A Path with Heart

If you can honestly say you love what you do, you are a very lucky person indeed. When you love your work, it ceases to be work. When you love your life, you find it so fascinating that you can't wait to jump out of bed in the morning for another day. It brings you pleasure, challenge, growth and fulfilment. Maybe you also derive self-esteem and a sense of identity through what you do, too. The hours you spend working are so much fun, it doesn't feel tiring.

You may be hoping to create just such a life. Perhaps you've had the courage to leave a boring humdrum job, or maybe you want to make the most out of being made redundant, or maybe you just want a new career. Suddenly you may face countless opportunities, unknown risks, and the loss of everything familiar. Following the steps in this book can help you find your way. However, the most important factor will always be to follow your Heart.

> *A path is only a path; if you feel you should not follow it, you must not stay with it under any conditions. But your decision to keep on the path or to leave it must be free of fear or ambition. All paths are the same: they lead nowhere. Before you embark on a path, ask the question: Does this path have a heart? If the answer is 'No' you will know it and then you must choose another path. A path without heart is never enjoyable. You have to work hard even to take it. On the other hand, a path with heart is easy; it does not make you work at liking it . . . .*
>
> Carlos Castaneda: *The Teachings of Don Juan*

After years of preparing to become a coach, one of my clients needed to rediscover the path of her Heart. She just couldn't take the final steps forward. Her inertia felt like being stuck in treacle. Instead of feeling excited about her new career, the middle of her chest felt like a heavy rock, dead and dull. Not surprisingly, she wasn't sure what her purpose was anymore, despite having many great ideas for different projects she wanted to undertake. Her fears were about not being good enough. 'How arrogant to think I could guide others!' The inertia of doing nothing felt so much more comfortable! She was also afraid her new career could possibly upset the balance of her marriage. All of these fears threatened to outweigh her real fascination and desire: to help people unleash their potential.

This heavy 'rock' she felt in her chest was keeping her safe, but limited. This part of her lacked courage, and wanted her to keep doing the stuff she knew how to do. This rock had appeared three years ago, just at the time when she became extremely bored with her previous job. She had become tired of doing the same things, bogged down in detail. Although there was an opportunity to take that project to a whole new level, she didn't feel she knew how to do it. More importantly, she didn't want to! So she had resigned. She realised that what had been driving her in that job was a sense that 'if she didn't do it, she would let herself down'. In fact, this was a hidden 'Have to'. Although the job had felt exciting when she first got it, over the years, she had outgrown it. Now her Heart wasn't in it anymore.

But was her Heart excited about the new projects she was contemplating? Her head came up with all kinds of logical, reasonable answers about how good each idea was. But which one was a true path of the Heart? She had forgotten to tune into her feelings. When she focused on how she was feeling in her Heart, at first it felt too small for its job, it was so full of fear and confusion. There was a bit of conflict, and even some hysteria, but as she gave herself permission to feel all these feelings, they passed. Then she re-discovered her inner wisdom, calmness, energy and optimism. From a deep sense of inner wholeness she could feel what was real for her.

This was the only missing ingredient! Every one of her ideas and plans for her new projects were wonderful. All she needed to do was to tune in to her Heart regularly to make sure she was still following her true path. It is so easy to get seduced by thoughts of what you should do, or have to do, or can't do! But when you choose a path with Heart, it will sustain you with the sheer joy of doing it.

> *The miracle comes quietly into the mind that stops an instant and is still.*
>
> A Course in Miracles

Before you start manifesting your Dream Script, it's a good idea to check with your feelings and make sure that the direction you are choosing is a path with Heart. This is an important reminder to keep in touch with your feelings, and to practise listening to what your Heart has to say. Your feelings can help you stay true to your purpose, and avoid getting stuck in 'have tos', 'shoulds' or any other heady ideas. Remember that your feelings are the most reliable communication from the creative side of your mind.

Exercise: Choosing a path with Heart ....

Check with your feelings to be sure you are on the right path
1. Meditate, go for a walk in nature, do whatever will help you to clear your mind and access your Heart.
2. Be willing to just FEEL. Imagine you could just hold each feeling in your arms like a little baby. Listen to, respect and feel each emotion until the next one comes up.
3. Keep going until you reach a place of emptiness, where no more feelings appear. Feel the emptiness and keep going even deeper until you can finally access your deepest inner core – the real truth in your Heart – a positive, calm peaceful place that feels true.
4. From this perspective, think about your Dream Script. Is this a path with Heart?

....

Keeping Oneself Small

Have you ever noticed how some people actually take pains to avoid talking about how successful they are, or how good life is, for fear of sounding big headed? Instead they lower their voice and speak about what difficulties they have, the problems they face, and how hard they are working. Even a fantastic holiday is often downplayed and understated. Is this about modesty and humility or does it speak more about keeping oneself small? Perhaps it is an old habit that goes back to the idea of 'not stepping out of one's place'. It might also be an attempt to avoid boasting and sounding arrogant.

What about people who have a more balanced optimism and who cheerfully self-promote themselves in a non-offensive way? They seem to enjoy nothing better than to let you know what good things are happening in their lives. Can you take pleasure in revealing your personal good fortune? Do you bubble with happiness and good cheer? Or does complaining seem more intelligent, more real, more acceptable? Grumbling and complaining comments constitute the greatest part of many people's conversation. The weather is not good enough, travel is a problem, overcrowding, pollution, high prices, problems at work, problems at home, problems with children, health problems. The list of troubles people whinge about is endless. Unfortunately, complaining lowers everyone's energy by directing attention to what is wrong, rather than what is good. While there is a part of the mind that needs to protect your survival by spotting potential problems, complaining turns this into an art form. What's worse is that it generates little energy for finding solutions to these problems.

Have you ever noticed that when you complain, you feel a little indulgent? Of course, if you are complaining about something or someone else, then at least it deflects attention away from what might be wrong with you. It also is more likely to gain instant acceptance with others since the habit is so common. What makes you feel more comfortable, singing the praises of something or pointing out what is wrong with it? Does complaining serve any useful purpose? Especially in its worst form – nagging – it rarely inspires people to change. Complaining doesn't motivate people. Instead it just keeps flowing like an endless river of misery and woe, sapping the energy and breeding discouragement. It can be quite destructive. Complaining often masks anger and disappointment. Something or someone is not behaving according to your plan.

Your plans and expectations of how things should be, can be a double-edged sword. It is great to have high standards and positive goals to aspire to. But the difference between reality and your expectations causes more distress than anything else. If you think of expectations as a form of perfectionism, then it becomes easy to understand how you can feel disappointed and frustrated, when things don't meet the mark.

Oprah Winfrey tells a story about driving home with her husband. For years she told him to make the same right turn at a certain junction, so they could save four miles on their journey. She couldn't understand why he never remembered that she wanted to go that way! One day she finally asked him, and he told her that he preferred the other road, because of the beautiful, scenic view that he enjoyed sharing with her. When she realised that insisting on 'her way' had actually deprived them of some quality time together, she realised it was time to let go of her expectations of how she thought things should be.

Complaining is an important habit to break if you want to manifest your Dream Script into real life. One definition of insanity is to repeat the same behaviour again and again, but expect to achieve a different outcome. Even if you complain silently, or you only complain about your own shortcomings, it will not help you towards your Dream Script. Complaining is rarely listened to, appreciated, thanked, loved or admired as expert advice, nor does it produce change. It is just a bad habit. You can exude whinge energy just by a look or by how you walk into a room. So, be aware that your non-verbal messages might reveal any complaints that are running through your mind. There's no such thing as a private thought!

Sometimes complaining takes on a more universal flavour. When you complain about your whole life not being the way you want, or bad fate, bad luck, being hard done by, you direct your anger at everyone, life, God or the universe. Unfortunately this directs your energy away from remembering who you really are, who you came to be and what you came to do. So commit now to give up any indulgent habit you have about complaining. Stop telling stories about how bad everything is. Make the choice to focus your energy on your positive direction instead.

The cure for complaining is appreciating. Research has proved that people (and animals) respond much faster to reward than to punishment. When you praise someone, or appreciate what they do, or give them some kind of appropriate reward, they feel much more inclined to do more of that, and to do an even better job next time. My friend tells a story about how she always complained that her husband never helped with the washing up. Then one day, she 'caught' him doing the washing up. Astonished and delighted, she came up behind him and gave him a big juicy hug. Funnily enough, he was back in the kitchen doing the washing up every night from then on!

Exercise: Antidote to complaining..

1. First start becoming aware of how often you complain, and the varied forms that it takes. Catch yourself in the act.
2. Note down what you complain about most often: weather, work, health, relationships, children, transport, prices, food, prejudice, injustice, unfairness. Do you have favourite stories?
3. Notice the tone of voice you use when you complain, and get in touch with the feelings you have while you are complaining. Who do you sound like? What are all the feelings underneath?
4. What is the intention behind your message? Who are you really complaining to? Make a list of who you think is at fault.
5. Note down what you have been expecting to happen instead. What are your criteria and specifications in your perfect world? How realistic are your expectations?
6. What is the real purpose of this indulgence? What is it you are really wanting?
7. Once you know what you really want, find a creative way to start appreciating how you already have that. Notice how most of your needs and wants are being taken care of, although maybe not by the person you focus on. Catch people in the act of doing something good and reward them.
8. Start with an attitude of gratitude. Thank people for everything they do. Thank the world for being such a perfect place to learn such lessons. Thank life.

Gratitude

It might still seem like a funny idea, but the faster you can appreciate and feel grateful for whatever happens in your life, the faster you can turn it around. Although it may be hard to accept a situation that seems disastrous, the truth is that you don't know what will happen next, or as a result. You also don't know what worse things could have happened. If you hold onto the negative feelings and judgements, you will get stuck. But if you can trust that somehow whatever is happening can continue to help you in your purpose, you can heal and move on. When you remember to be grateful no matter what, you are free and open to make the best of whatever comes next. Ask yourself what resources, what gifts, and what experiences do I have right now to be grateful for, and what can I do with those? What can I learn from this experience? In what way does this challenge me to grow? What am I being called to do or be right now?

Curiosity

As well as being appreciative and grateful, having an attitude of curiosity will help you throughout your whole journey as you begin to manifest your Dream Script. Just imagine that everything that is happening right now in your life has some incredible part to play in making your dreams come true. If it didn't happen, then the next thing couldn't happen and so on and so forth. What if every person you meet has some important gift, some piece of knowledge, a reminder, an example or an inspiration that could help you? What if how you interact with each person is a vital factor in developing your true self? What if how you respond to everything and every detail is crucial to your success? Wouldn't you become more curious to just experience everything and watch the whole process unfold? How does what has happened in the past, what is happening now, and what will happen in the future, all relate? Being curious to find out could make your journey much more interesting.

I want to beg you, as much as I can, to be patient toward
all that is unresolved in your heart and try to love the
questions themselves like the locked rooms and like books

that are written in a very foreign tongue. Do not seek the answers, which cannot be given to you because you would not be able to live them. And the point is to live everything. Live the questions now. Perhaps you will then gradually without noticing it, live along some distant day into the answer.

Rainer Maria Rilke

Be curious about how your whole life could be the answer to your inner purpose, rather than being too quick to analyse and categorise everything. Resist the urge to put things in boxes and think that your judgements are the truth. Once again, allow some flexibility, some mystery, some space for different endings. There could be better outcomes to your story than the ones you may have imagined. Your Dream Script might develop into something the world has never seen before!

Apprentice Yourself to a Master

When you were a child, you learned how to do things by watching everyone around you. You watched how your parents did things, and then you copied them. You learned how to talk by making the same sounds you heard your parents speak, and you unconsciously learned a great deal about the world through their unspoken beliefs and their way of handling situations. Modelling other people is still the fastest way to learn new skills and to achieve excellence. During the Renaissance, apprentices worked with the old masters to learn their craft. Similarly, you could gain valuable expertise by interviewing, and working with people who already excel at what you want to do. Where could you go to meet these people? Who could you model that could give you useful tips, advice and actually show you how to succeed in your Dream Script?

If you could learn how to be like them, if you could walk, talk, stand, breathe and do things the way they do, you could learn the essence of what works for them. Then, after you have mastered that, you could make it your own and add your own flavour and style. Another way to do this is to imagine the 'you' of the future, already successfully living your Dream Script to the full. How would this future you walk, talk, breathe and dress your purpose? How would you be giving your gifts? In every little thing you do, how would you be behaving differently? How much energy can you put into this? The more you can breathe life into this new way of being, the easier it will become to start living your Dream Script right now.

Your imagination is your preview of life's coming attractions.
Albert Einstein

Most successful people share the ability to manage their emotional state. What sets them apart from others is not that they are more talented, or more gifted, but that they have learned helpful ways to respond to any situation. Instead of reacting in anger, fear, or on impulse, they stop to breathe and respond intelligently. While noting the positive intentions behind what is going on, they never lose sight of their direction. They look to learn from each mistake and turn it around as fast as possible. They stay as flexible as a dancer while looking for new solutions to get back on track. But more than anything, they enjoy every moment of the whole process.

Remember to breathe and ask yourself:
- What is not perfect yet for achieving my purpose and direction?
- How could what is happening have a positive intention?
- Can I remember who I am and enjoy the journey?
- What will help me be flexible in finding new solutions?
- Why not have fun doing whatever it takes to succeed?

Who is on Your Team?
You might think that your life is all about what you do, how well you perform and how creative you might be. The truth is, however, that successful people never work all alone. They are the first ones to appreciate that many people have supported them to make what they do possible. They acknowledge all the learning, insight and inspiration they have gained from people who travelled before them. They know that they stand on the

shoulders of others. They also know that the support of their family, friends and colleagues has been essential to their success.

Who is on your team in your Dream Script? Who already supports you and encourages you? Can you identify all the people who are helpful to you in some important way? When you appreciate how many people have already contributed to your life, you may begin to realise how connected you are to your own personal network. Be grateful for all the support you have received, and all the lessons you have learned from others.

Before you use the Manifesting Exercise, please double check that each of the goals in your Dream Script meets the following criteria. If you have carefully followed the exercises throughout the previous chapters, these requirements should already be met.

Review each goal of your Dream Script:

- You must believe it is possible.
- You must be willing to do whatever it takes to make it happen, including changing old habits of thinking and behaving.
- You must let go of doubt.
- You must let go of obsessively wanting it too much.
- You must let go of expectations about exactly how it should be.
- You must forgive yourself and others for any past mistakes.
- You must clear out hidden needs and intentions.
- You must appreciate, understand and respect and give yourself permission to feel anger, guilt, fear or other negative emotions.
- You must give up complaining and negative self talk.
- You must have an attitude of gratitude towards everything in your life.

When you feel that you *deserve* to have everything in your Dream Script, just as naturally as you deserve to breathe, or to grow, then you are ready to manifest it.

Exercise: Manifesting your Dream Script.............................

When you are ready, here are the final steps to making your dreams into reality!

1. Get into a relaxed state, in a place where you will be undisturbed.
2. Imagine yourself living your Dream Script in full colour, sound and feelings. Imagine you could step into it and experience it fully as if it was happening now. When is this future 'now'? Note the time and date.
3. Step out, leaving a clone image of yourself still living the movie of your Dream Script.
4. As you continue to watch the movie, breathe and send all your energy to that whole story, remembering how good it will feel to be giving your gifts and living your purpose fully. Then let that go for a moment.
5. Relax and think about some event that you know with absolute *certainty* is going to happen in the near future. It can be anything you are certain will happen.
6. As you think about this event, notice a picture you make of it in your mind. Notice the qualities of that picture. Quickly circle the answers to the following questions:
   Is the picture a movie or still shot?
   Is it panoramic or in a frame?
   Is it in colour or black and white?
   What kind of colour – normal or muted?
   Where is the picture located – right in front of you, up or down, or to the right or left?
   How far away is the picture – close up, arms length, distant?
   Do you see your body in the picture?
   Is it in sharp focus or fuzzy or vague?
   Is there sound?
   Are there any body sensations?
   Are there any feelings?
7. Put your attention back on your Dream Script movie picture. Look at that picture carefully.
8. Adjust the qualities of your Dream Script movie picture to have all the same qualities as the ones you have circled in question 6. Notice if it starts to feel more possible or certain.
9. Trust that this Dream Script can now happen as easily as that other event that you just imagined.
10. The most important step: LET IT GO. Just trust that events will now unfold to help you create the life of your dreams.

Forget about getting to the finish line. Instead focus on enjoying the process of going towards your true direction. Make the most of whatever happens.

....

Measuring Your Success

If you are letting go of your Dream Script and trusting that it will now happen, at what point is it appropriate to check on its progress? How will you be able to measure your success, or know when it might be necessary to make some adjustments? It could be crucial to check whether or not things are going according to plan. Make a note of when some positive results should begin appearing in your life. Choose some time markers as check points. Although the journey to any kind of success often follows a zigzag path, there should be some signs that things are progressing well. But even if a situation looks disastrous, you can never tell how events might unfold to bring you what you asked for in surprisingly different ways.

If you think that nothing has changed at all, and the same old script seems to be running, then it is time to do a re-assessment. Perhaps you have missed some important factor. Maybe something else requires your attention and understanding. There could be some more forgiveness necessary before your path to success is clear. Review each section and re-do the exercises to find out what you might have missed before. Make some better choices.

When you are so happy enjoying your journey, and fascinated with the unfolding process of your life that you forget about whether or not your Dream Script is working out, chances are it will surprise you by happening almost effortlessly. Here are some final checkpoints to help you live the life of your dreams:

- Maintain your curiosity and flexibility about how it will unfold.
- Enjoy the process of moving towards your goals more than getting the final results. Be in each moment as much as possible.
- Take full responsibility for whatever happens, and respond as if everything that happens is part of your plan.

- Make the best of whatever happens and keep moving towards your true direction and purpose.
- Let go and forget about focusing on getting results.
- Have trust and certainty that everything that is true for you will happen.

Letting Go

Letting go of your Dream Script might seem strange to you after spending so much time creating it and exploring it. But letting go is the most crucial factor for success. You must let go of your expectations, let go of your need to have it, let go of your desire for immediate results, let go of your deadlines, and let go of your plan for how things should be. Only then do you allow the universe the freedom to deliver even more extraordinary ways for your Dream Script to manifest.

Trust that it will happen with full certainty. Continue to act as if you are the star in your Dream Script, and focus all your energy on your purpose and your positive long-term direction. Be neither optimistic nor pessimistic, neither high nor low. Make no comparisons between where you are now and where you might want to be. Reframe any negative thought or doubt that might try to creep into your awareness. Just keep trusting and stepping forward – you are already in the opening frames of your movie. The fastest way to manifest miracles is to make the best of each moment now and enjoy absolutely everything. Keep doing whatever will take you in the direction you want to go.

There is only one time when it is essential to awaken. That time is now.

Buddha

An Easy Path

By following the steps throughout this book, you will have experienced an extraordinary journey. Between designing a Dream Script for your life and learning how to make it a reality, there have been many stops along the way. Each digression offered you opportunities to view the passing scenery differently.

Connecting with your Heart kept you firmly grounded. Remembering your gifts, your goals and your Purpose gave you support. You learned how to tread carefully around hidden needs, fears, and intentions. You looked back at the past and discovered new ways to let go and forgive. When there were conflicts about which direction to take, I hope you chose the path with Heart.

Learning these skills and techniques for the first time paves the way for future journeys. You will find that you can speed up the pace. You'll be able to skip through many of the exercises quickly as you become more familiar with what is true for you. Soon you'll surprise yourself by manifesting things in moments! Remember the easy way forward will always be to follow your Heart. Enjoy your journey!

Resources and Recommended Reading

Resources
For details about:

- Workshops in *Compassionate Coaching* Techniques
- Arielle Essex's Meditation CDs for Healing, Relaxation, Pain Relief etc.
- Private sessions with Arielle Essex
- Practitioner Trainings in Neuro Linguistic Programming
- Talks, newsletters and products

please contact:
Practical Miracles
Website: www.practicalmiracles.com
E-mail: info@practicalmiracles.com
12 Prince of Wales Mansions
Prince of Wales Drive
London SW11 4BG
020 7622 4670

Recommended Reading

Steve Andreas and Charles Faulkner, *NLP: The New Technology of Achievement* (Nicholas Brealey, 1996).

Anon, *A Course in Miracles* (Penguin Arkana, 1975).

Coleman Barks (trans.) with John Moyne, *The Essential Rumi* (Castle Books, 1997).

Richard Carlson PhD and Benjamin Shield (eds.), *Healers on Healing* (Jeremy P. Tarcher, 1989).

Doc Childre and Howard Martin, *The Heartmath Solution* (Piatkus Books, 1999).

Deepak Chopra, *Quantum Healing* (Bantam Books, 1989).

Deepak Chopra, *Unconditional Life* (Bantam Books, 1991).

Norman Cousins, *Headfirst: The Biology of Hope and the Healing Power of the Human Spirit* (Penguin Books, 1989).

Robert Dilts, Tim Hallbom and Suzi Smith, *Beliefs* (Metamorphous Press, 1990).

Robert Fritz, *The Path of Least Resistance* (Fawcett Columbine, 1984).

Steve Gilligan, *The Courage to Love* (W.W. Norton and Co, 1997).

Daniel Goleman, *Emotional Intelligence* (Bloomsbury, 1996).

Miranda Holden, *Boundless Love* (Rider, 2002).

Robert Holden, *Happiness Now* (Hodder & Stoughton, 1998).

Tad James and Wyatt Woodsmall, *Time Line Therapy* (Meta Publications, Cupertino, 1988).

Serge King, *Mastering Your Hidden Self* (Quest Books, 1985).

Sue Knight, *NLP at Work – NLP Solutions* (Nicholas Brealey, 1999).

Barbara Levine, *Your Body Believes Every Word You Say* (Aslan Publishing, 1991).

Byron A. Lewis and Frank Pucelik, *Magic of NLP Demystified* (Metamorphous Press, 1982).

Niro Markoff Asistent, *Why I Survived AIDS* (Fireside/Simon & Schuster, 1991).

Caroline Myss, *Anatomy of the Spirit* (Bantam, 1997).

Caroline Myss, *Why People Don't Heal and How They Can* (Bantam 1997).

Nick Owen, *The Magic of Metaphor* (Crownhouse, 2001).

Anthony Robbins, *Unlimited Power* (Simon & Schuster, 1997).

Anthony Robbins, *Awaken the Giant Within* (Simon & Schuster, 1991).

John Roger and Peter McWilliams, *You Can't Afford the Luxury of a Negative Thought* (Prelude Press, 1991).

Debbie Shapiro, *The BodyMind WorkBook* (Piatkus, 1996).

Debbie Shapiro, *Your Body Speaks Your Mind* (Piatkus 1996).

Sidney and Suzanne Simon, *Forgiveness* (Warner Books, 1990).

Chuck Spezzano, *50 Ways to Let Go and Be Happy* (Coronet, 2001).

Chuck Spezzano, *If it Hurts It Isn't Love* (Hodder & Stoughton, 1999).

Lency Spezzano, *Make Way for Love* (Psychology of Vision Press, 1996).

Colin C. Tipping, *Radical Forgiveness* (Gill and MacMillan, 2000).

Eckhart Tolle, The Power of Now (Hodder & Stoughton, 1999).

Dr Thomas Verney with John Kelly, *The Secret Life of the Unborn Child* (Sphere Books, 1982).

Nick Williams, *The Work We Were Born to Do* (Element, 1999).

Marianne Williamson, *A Return to Love* (Harper Collins, 1992).

Paramahansa Yogananda, *Autobiography of a Yogi* (Rider Books, 1996).

THE ROAD LESS TRAVELLED

A New Psychology of Love, Traditional Values
and Spiritual Growth

M. Scott Peck
Author of the bestseller
The Road Less Travelled and Beyond

Confronting and solving problems is a painful process that most of us attempt to avoid. And the very avoidance results in greater pain and an inability to grow both mentally and spiritually. Drawing heavily on his own professional experience, Dr M. Scott Peck, a psychiatrist, suggests ways in which facing our difficulties – and suffering through the changes – can enable us to reach a higher level of self-understanding. He discusses the nature of loving relationships: how to recognise true compatibility; how to distinguish dependency from love; how to become one's own person and how to be a more sensitive parent.

This book can show you how to embrace reality and yet achieve serenity and a richer existence. Hugely influential, it has now sold over 7 million copies – and has changed many people's lives round the globe. It may change yours.

'Magnificent . . . this is not just a book but a spontaneous act of generosity written by an author who leans towards the reader for the purpose of sharing something larger than himself.'   – *Washington Post*

THE HEART OF LEADERSHIP

Unlock Your Inner Wisdom, and Inspire Others

Sabina Spencer

We stand in the doorway of the Relationship Age, says Sabina Spencer. With rapid connections now possible through the internet and digital technology, we feel the links between us more strongly than ever before. Words like 'networks', 'alliances', 'partnerships' and 'communities' reflect our sense of connection and require a very different orientation to leadership. We can no longer operate with a divide and conquer mentality, putting self-interest above the common good.

In this groundbreaking book, the author explains that there are seven keys we need to possess if we want to be a source of inspiration to others. And once we have mastered these, we will be able to create a future that is enriching and sustainable for everyone.

'Read this book if you are prepared to broaden yourself and your leadership approach beyond what you previously thought was possible.'
– Phil Hodgson, Director of Leadership Programmes, Ashridge Management College

'This brilliant book provides an inspiring vision as well as practical ideas and tools that will help anyone interested in being an effective leader and a fulfilled human being.'
– Shakti Gawain, author of *Creative Visualisation*

BOUNDLESS LOVE

Transforming Your Life with Grace and Inspiration

Miranda Holden

In *Boundless Love*, Miranda Holden shows us how to create a freer, more inspired life – one filled with deep joy and a sense of connection. Writing about some of our most important concerns, she shares rich insights gleaned from her own personal challenges, intuitive wisdom and extensive study into spirituality, grace and transformation.

Full of encouraging stories, meditations and spiritual practices, this challenging yet compassionate book explains how to:

- Connect with your heart's deepest yearnings
- Go direct to God
- Reclaim timeless wisdom
- Cultivate a deep sense of calm
- Heal your blocks to love
- Illuminate daily life
- Achieve a powerful breakthrough

Read it and transform your life.

'Pure spiritual medicine for modern times. Take this book to heart and let it change your life.'
         – Paul Wilson, author of *The Little Book of Calm*

THE GOOD RETREAT GUIDE

Over 500 Places to Find Peace and Spiritual Renewal
in Britain, Ireland, France, Spain and Greece

Stafford Whiteaker

The Good Retreat Guide is the definitive work on where
to find a retreat that suits you. This popular book is sought
out by busy people living a hectic lifestyle – everyone
in fact who needs to find a place where the noise and
stress of the world will not intrude – somewhere that
nurtures your spirit and returns you home refreshed.
Whatever your beliefs, Europe's most authoritative
guide offers the greatest choice of retreats, explaining the
different types of retreat available and how to find the
best one for you.

'A flip through its pages is an eye-opening experience.'
                                    – *Sunday Telegraph*

'Deservedly popular and very helpful.'
                                    – *Yoga and Health*

'The definitive guide.'

                                    – *Marie Claire*